"What a wonderful book. Everything y(
last is someone writing with real experier
with playgroups, and treating children wit
researched both the traditional Chinese ι
practical advice and delicious recipes that are actually possible for a busy
mother or father to cook."

—Dr Julian Scott, PhD, Cert Ac (and family cook!)

"As a practitioner of Chinese Medicine, I have always focused on the
importance of diet and lifestyle with all of my patients, including the
children I treat. Sandra Robertson covers and explains all the important areas
of Chinese nutrition, including foods for common childhood conditions,
and foods that are beneficial during the different seasons, and she gives lots
of wonderful recipes. She fills a very big gap in the practice of pediatrics in
Chinese Medicine, and has created a user-friendly book for practitioners
and for parents to help them establish a good foundation for their children's
health. I love this book and will use it and recommend it!"

—Deirdre Courtney, MTCM, author of
Nourishing Life the Yang Sheng Way

"*Treating Children with Chinese Dietary Therapy* is a much-needed book,
bursting with useful information and tasty recipes. It skillfully brings
together ancient Chinese Medicine wisdom and modern research and will
be of great value to parents and to practitioners working with children."

—Rebecca Avern, BA (Hons), Lic Ac, Dip Paed, senior faculty member at
the College of Integrated Chinese Medicine and author of
Acupuncture for Babies, Children and Teenagers

"Due to the huge differences between Chinese and Western cultures and
languages, as well as the breadth and depth of Traditional Chinese Medicine,
it is difficult to accurately express its theories and methods in English;
Sandra has managed to do this. Capturing its essence with accurate and
effective advice for children's dietary therapy, I think this is a great reference
book for parents and practitioners."

—Dr Ganglin Yin, Principal of Oshio College of Acupuncture and
Herbology (Victoria, BC, Canada), and author of
Three Needle Technique *and* Advanced Modern
Chinese Acupuncture Therapy

Treating Children with Chinese Dietary Therapy

Sandra Robertson

Foreword by Lillian Pearl Bridges

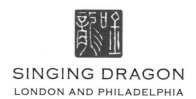

SINGING DRAGON
LONDON AND PHILADELPHIA

First published in Great Britain in 2021 by Singing Dragon,
an imprint of Jessica Kingsley Publishers
An Hachette Company

3

Copyright © Sandra Robertson 2021
Foreword copyright © Lillian Pearl Bridges 2021

Excerpts from *The Yellow Emperor's Classic of Medicine*, translated and with commentary
by Maoshing Ni, © 1995 by Maoshing Ni. Reprinted by arrangement with The Permissions
Company, LLC on behalf of Shambhala Publications Inc., Boulder, Colorado, shambhala.com.

Excerpts from *Healing with Whole Foods: Asian Traditions and Modern Nutrition, Third
Edition* by Paul Pitchford, published by North Atlantic Books, copyright © 1993,1996,
2002 by Paul Pitchford. Reprinted by permission of North Atlantic Books.

The epigraph on p.158 is taken from the book *The Tao of Motherhood*.
Copyright © 1997 Vimala McClure. Reprinted with permission of New
World Library, Novato, CA, www.newworldlibrary.com.

Front cover image source: Shutterstock®. The cover image is for
illustrative purposes only, and any person featuring is a model.

Disclaimer: The information contained in this book is not intended to replace
the services of trained medical professionals or to be a substitute for medical
advice. The complementary therapy described in this book may not be suitable for
everyone to follow. You are advised to consult a doctor before embarking on any
complementary therapy program and on any matters relating to your health, and
in particular on any matters that may require diagnosis or medical attention.

A CIP catalogue record for this title is available from the
British Library and the Library of Congress

ISBN 978 1 78775 318 1
eISBN 978 1 78775 319 8

Printed and bound by CPI Group (UK) Ltd, Croydon, CR0 4YY

Jessica Kingsley Publishers' policy is to use papers that are natural, renewable and recyclable
products and made from wood grown in sustainable forests. The logging and manufacturing
processes are expected to conform to the environmental regulations of the country of origin.

Jessica Kingsley Publishers
Carmelite House
50 Victoria Embankment
London EC4Y 0DZ

www.singingdragon.com

Contents

Foreword

What a wonderful gift this book is for parents and parents-to-be! It's chock-full of advice about how to feed children starting in the womb and into childhood in the best possible ways. I would have loved to have owned this book and used it as a reference when my children were still at home. I'm definitely going to be giving them a copy now that they have children of their own.

Sandra Robertson was a student of mine at my school, the Lotus Institute, studying Facial Diagnosis in my Master Face Reading Certification Program. From the beginning, it was very clear that she was particularly interested in working with children and we had many discussions about how to apply Facial Diagnosis to her young patients. She then very systematically tested the diagnostic criteria she learned in comparison to their Western Diagnoses. I was very taken with her dedication to treating children and I encouraged her to write this book.

While I learned many of the principles of Chinese Medicine from my Chinese mother and her family, it was often hard to remember what was best for them when they showed certain symptoms. Like all mothers, it is so helpful to have access to the wisdom of those who came before us. This book helps us remember to use natural food remedies as the first and often the best treatment for common childhood ailments.

Sandra has done a wonderful job taking the experience from her work as a Chinese medicine practitioner, along with her ongoing studies in the field, and she combines that with her own personal experience as a mother. Her approach in treating children with dietary therapy is presented in a fresh and creative way that is completely applicable to the modern lifestyle, while supported by scientific research.

Treating Children with Chinese Dietary Therapy is a comprehensive look at the nutritional needs of children, with wonderful tips to tempt them to eat healthfully. She covers many of the fundamental principles of Chinese Medicine that will help parents understand how to balance their children's lives and their diets. Even those people who are already familiar with Chinese Medicine can learn some important things from this book.

She covers the Chinese understanding of the temperature of foods and cooking methods and gives an overview of the five elements of food and flavor. She also covers the very important concept of eating with the seasons. The Chinese dietary principles are accompanied by a thorough listing of the vitamin and mineral content of foods, and she also gives vital information about how to help your child create a healthy microbiome. I was particularly taken with what she calls the "Color Food Game," which is a wonderful way of getting children involved in their own meal planning. She wisely encourages food positivity, which is something that I know is so needed for creating lifelong healthy eating habits.

I love her down-to-earth advice on how to manage a child's craving for sweet foods and how to feed them naturally sweet foods instead of processed and refined variations. This is something I definitely could have used as a mother! She thoroughly explains the effects of different foods on the delicate and somewhat immature digestive systems of children.

This book is a wonderful melding of Eastern dietary therapy and Western food science. It is full of ancient wisdom still applicable and necessary today. Sandra gives practical and helpful advice on taking care of children's health naturally with good food remedies and a balanced lifestyle. The bonus is the many delicious recipes that I'm quite sure kids will love.

What started as a desire to share what she learned from her own experience as a mother and as a practitioner of Chinese Medicine has culminated in this much-needed book. I'm so pleased to see the end result. I believe that every parent and grandparent should have a copy of this book!

Lillian Pearl Bridges, author of *Face Reading in Chinese Medicine* and *Divine Chinese Cuisine*

Introduction

Parents want the best for their children. This is a universal truth. They want them to be happy, successful, healthy, and resilient. They want them to be robust so they can focus on learning, playing, thriving in school, playing sports, and enjoying hobbies. They do everything, from showering them with love, to making sure they are taking vitamins, to signing them up for creative lessons, to using positive phrasing, and to trying to feed them as healthy a diet as possible. The list could go on and on as there are many books and lots of information out there, educating parents on every possible facet of parenting, as well as leading-edge research guiding them on how to raise their children in the best way possible.

It can be overwhelming and confusing to sort through this mountain of parental advice, particularly in regard to diet and nutrition. Parents have a lot of questions around what and when and how to feed their children. While Traditional Chinese Medicine (TCM) dietary therapy is based on sound principles that are practical and make good sense, the principles, sadly, are not commonly understood or known outside the community of Chinese medical practitioners, partly because food therapy instruction is usually only given out to help bring about healing from an illness. It is so much more than that, though; it is a way of eating that strives to maintain a state of feeling well, a way of eating that PREVENTS illness and strives for long-term health benefits.

Our current generation of children is being called "Generation RX" because of all the health concerns they are experiencing, and the alarmingly high rates of pharmaceuticals being prescribed. Doctors are quick to prescribe them because they are a quick fix, but they are most often neither beneficial in the long run nor holistic. Our Western mentality of overusing antibiotics has led to antibiotic resistance and super bugs. Corticosteroids are readily prescribed for asthma and allergies, but come with side effects. When children develop food sensitivities, we take away the offending food instead of looking deeper into the imbalance in the body that may be the cause. These are the band aid treatments that will, unfortunately, only create more sickness, disease, and imbalance.

There is much controversy and debate over what we should and should not eat. For a long time, we were told that fat was considered the enemy and should be removed from our diets—eat it and you would end up with arteries that resembled New York traffic jams. Now we know that healthy fats (butter, olive oil, eggs, nuts, seeds, fish, grass-fed beef) are a major source of energy in the body and help us to absorb vitamins and minerals. This is the same for children and adults alike. Most of us have grown up far removed from the farm where food is grown, and we take it for granted that all vegetables and fruits are available year-round at the grocery store. We also don't give ourselves enough time to really taste the different qualities and flavors of food, often eating on the run or in front of the television.

I was first introduced to Chinese dietary therapy in my early 20s when I started my studies on Chinese Medicine. I was suffering from Irritable Bowel Syndrome (IBS), a common disorder that affects the large intestine. Symptoms are usually cramping, abdominal pain, bloating, gas, diarrhea and/or constipation. As I learned the concepts of Chinese dietary therapy, I gradually shifted the way I cooked—what I ate, when to include certain foods and when to omit them—and focused on stoking my digestive fire to keep my Middle Burner strong. The IBS resolved and hasn't shown up for 20 years.

One of the most effective ways in which we can help children is through what we feed them. In the East, diet and health are, and have always been, synonymous. As much as this concept is understood in the West, our idea of a "healthy diet" doesn't include strengthening the digestion, which is at the core of what Chinese dietary therapy is all about. This is why I wanted to write a book on Chinese dietetics solely focused on children, to give Chinese medicine practitioners and other holistic practitioners a resource to bring this ancient awareness to today's parents.

The guiding principles of TCM, once shared and applied, could change countless lives. If children grow up with a strong digestion, they will be much more resilient and have better immune systems. They will be much more connected to how they feel after eating a certain way, and will be more likely to make better food choices for themselves as they become teenagers.

Why don't we give children a solid health foundation using wisdom that has been around for thousands of years? Many books have been written on dietary therapy in the long history of TCM. The earliest existing Chinese dietary text is a chapter of Sun Simiao's *Prescriptions Worth a Thousand in Gold*, written in the Tang dynasty in 650. He wrote that, "people who practice medicine must first thoroughly understand the source of the disorder and know what has been violated. Then, use food to treat it, and if food will not cure it, afterwards apply drugs" (quoted in Wilms 2010). In the 1300s, Hu Sihui wrote the *Principles of Correct Diet*, the first dietary manual in Chinese history. It included information on eating in moderation, using variety in one's diet, proper hygiene, and food storage, and using special diets for pregnant women and children. His book describes how some diseases can be connected to dietary deficiencies. It is considered a classic in TCM and cuisine, and its relevance is shown by still being in print in China today.

How often do our healthcare providers ask if we, or our children, are eating a nutritionally balanced and digestive-enhancing diet before being prescribed medicine? It takes one hospital visit in the West to realize that we have not yet caught up with understanding the importance of a truly wholesome and nourishing meal. Jell-O®, which is mainly sugar and dye, is still routinely served for sick and recovering patients. Sugar-sweetened fruit juice and yoghurt, frosted flakes, mushy vegetables, and iceberg lettuce are some other rather nonnutritive menu options.

As a licensed practitioner of Chinese Medicine, I have, over the last 15 years, practiced and studied its intricacies and have treated thousands of patients in my clinic in Victoria, BC, Canada. I will almost always ask about or advise on diet, and I have been able to adjust what and how my clients eat to bring about healing.

Why children's dietary therapy?

The information in this book is focused on children for a few different reasons. First, when I had originally searched for children's dietary therapy from a TCM viewpoint, I couldn't find a whole book on the subject. There are many books on the topic of Chinese dietary therapy, but none geared towards babies' and children's growing bodies.

Second, as the mother of two stepsons and a daughter, I have had to make breakfasts, lunches, dinners, organize snacks, and think about this topic for the last 12 years. My knowledge, education, and experience as a TCM practitioner gave me a unique viewpoint at mealtimes. It taught me what to include and, more importantly, what to exclude. In the past I've also worked with preschool and kindergarten children, and was able to have a close look at what children were eating and drinking for lunch and snack time. Often "healthy" food given to the child was contributing to their runny nose, eczema, etc., and it was these times that I realized the role Chinese dietary therapy could have in prevention. Because China is a huge country with many different ethnic groups and varying climates from region to region, Chinese dietary therapy has been proven to work in a diverse group of people and climates, so it is easy to take the founding principles and adapt them to any geographical region.

I have always felt grateful to have this base of knowledge to help guide me through meal preparation for my children from babyhood and on. Every medical tradition recognizes the importance of early childhood health and wellness and the far-reaching, long-lasting effects it has on a child for the rest of their lives. They are a clean slate.

Lastly, adult health is laid down in infancy and childhood. The health of the pregnant mother and the time in the womb also plays a vital role. The healthier a child is, the more they can focus on learning and discovering their individual talents and strengths they bring into the world. Chinese dietary therapy can help to strengthen their immune system, help relieve constipation and diarrhea, decrease or eliminate skin problems like eczema, help prevent obesity, stop the lingering runny nose and a cough that don't seem to go away fully, and support appetite. Adults could have avoided many negative health conditions and unnecessary dieting had we been given this foundation. In my practice as a TCM practitioner I see many clients whose illnesses as adults (asthma, allergies, fatigue, diabetes, IBS, etc.) started to manifest when they were children. I know when I was growing up in the 1980s and 1990s I thought it was perfectly normal to microwave Tater Tots®, dip them into large dollops of ketchup and mayonnaise, and slurp down a coke slushy from the 7 Eleven store. Yikes, talk about sugar overload! I didn't realize the consequences that sitting on cold concrete and eating ice cream during menstruation could have in creating disharmony and pain during my monthly cycle; this cold evil over time invades the uterus and can cause pain and stagnation. While studying at a university hospital in Changsha, China, I spent my days with three different Chinese student female translators. They were all aware of the outcomes cold food or environment could have on a women's menstrual cycle; this is common knowledge in their culture passed along by parents and grandparents. I wasn't ever taught to think about what season it was and how I was going to keep myself warm internally through the winter or keep cool in the summer. As I started to learn and understand the concepts of TCM, my own personal habits and diet evolved and, as a result, I have become a much healthier and happier adult.

Traditional Chinese Medicine dietary therapy

TCM involves the use of many different healing techniques, such as acupuncture, herbal remedies, acupressure, Tui na, massage, Tai Chi, Qi Gong, and dietary therapy. Dietary therapy is used in place of medication for wellness and for disease prevention. The idea of dietary therapy is to strive for a balance in the five flavors: sweet, salty, pungent, bitter, and sour. Our Western culture is often too high on the sweet and salty scale and often lacking in the bitter and sour flavors. There isn't the understanding that sweet applies just as much to sugar as it does to sweet potatoes, oats, and almonds, for example. TCM classifies foods as having a warming, cooling, hot, cold, or neutral effect on the body. Foods can also be damp-forming, drying, astringing, or moistening. Certain foods can help stimulate the appetite, resolve phlegm, or soothe indigestion. And now we know that certain foods (prebiotics) feed our beneficial bacteria.

The earliest written record of TCM, the *Neijing* (*Inner Classic*) was written about 2500 years ago. This classical book goes into depth on topics about the nature of health, disease, and treatment. One of the resounding messages of these ancient writings is living in accordance with the world around us, the seasons, and listening to our intuition and our bodies. This means adjusting our diets seasonally, dressing appropriately, and altering how we cook our food. TCM shifts the way we look at food, so we don't just think in terms of calories and vitamins but, instead, about how and when and why to eat, and cook foods in certain ways. It's about bringing an attitude of joy and positivity to mealtimes, and cooking and eating with the idea of nourishing and balancing. If we can teach our children that food is medicine, they will hopefully start to trust their own judgment in knowing what they need to eventually make health-promoting food choices on their own.

Why include recent research into the gut microbiome?

TCM must have had some understanding of gut bacteria back in the 4th century. Dr Ge Hong, a physician in the Jin dynasty, would serve a broth consisting of a dried or fermented stool from a healthy person to someone suffering from diarrhea as a cure. As unsavory as this may sound—and it is not something I recommend trying—the goal was to incorporate healthy bacteria into the sick individual to promote healing 1700 years ago! Nowadays fecal microbiota transplantations (FMTs) are done to transfer the fecal matter from a donor to the intestinal tract of a recipient to confer a health benefit. I have included a chapter to discuss the importance of these microbes that are with us from the moment we are born (see Chapter 4). It is another reason to create a hospitable environment internally so that the beneficial bacteria (associated with health promotion) can be abundant and diverse and help to prevent colonization in the gut by harmful bacteria. This research ties into what TCM has always known—that our digestion is at the root of many health conditions.

Knowledge of the human microbiome broadened our understanding immensely after the five-year-long Human Microbiome Project (HMP), an international effort to characterize the microbial communities found in the human body and to identify each microorganism's role in health and disease. I've found this research fascinating, and it gives a scientific basis to the adage "you are what you eat." What makes it even more fascinating is that this microbial community is established in the first few years of life, so parents need to be aware of what can upset the natural balance and what will help the body to thrive.

Whether someone is vegan, vegetarian, or gluten-free, to name but a few, the knowledge in TCM will be the missing link to understanding the importance of digestive health, and it is able to offer a different viewpoint of what it means to nourish and bring the body closer to a state of balance and further from disease. There are ways for everyone to incorporate TCM dietary therapy into a child's life (and yours) no matter what your eating style is.

By the end of this book you will have become acquainted with the understanding that children's digestion has a pivotal role in sustaining and optimizing their health.

COVID-19

While writing this book (in 2020), the world around us as we once knew it has been transformed; a virus shut down our everyday lives and spread around the globe within months. I had to close my practice, as did millions of others in different professions and business establishments. It left many people feeling vulnerable, scared, and worried about the future and our loved ones. We can only be grateful that children have been mostly spared from encountering the worst of the virus and the intense version that adults seem to get. If it did not matter to us before, 2020 is surely a wake-up call to do all that we can to maintain sound health and a robust immune system. We are still living amid the pandemic as I write this, and we do not yet know what the outcome will be, but my hope is for the world to reassess what is important in life. In the words of Mahatma Gandhi,

It is health that is real wealth and not pieces of gold and silver.

A note on recipe measurements

I have used Canadian cup measurements for recipes throughout the book. I have provided a helpful table below outlining imperial to metric conversions, and for specific ingredient conversions into grams the following website may be useful: https://foodconverter.com

Imperial	Metric
⅛ tsp	0.5 ml
¼ tsp	1 ml
½ tsp	2.5 ml
1 tsp	5 ml
1 tbsp	15 ml
2 tbsp	30 ml
¼ cup	60 ml
⅓ cup	80 ml
½ cup	125 ml
⅔ cup	160 ml
¾ cup	180 ml
1 cup	250 ml

If you need assistance converting oven temperatures, please refer to the table that follows.

Celsius	Fahrenheit	Gas
140	275	1
150	300	2
170	325	3

cont.

Celsius	Fahrenheit	Gas
180	350	4
190	375	5
200	400	6
220	425	7
230	450	8

Acknowledgments

Thank you to my friend and teacher Lillian Pearl Bridges, who saw the writer in me and assured me I could write this book. I am forever grateful to you for your insight and teachings. A huge thank you to Claire Wilson, my commissioning editor, for turning this dream of a book into a reality. Many thanks to the team at Singing Dragon, specifically Claire Robinson and Maddy Budd for all your help and professionalism; you were a joy to collaborate with.

Thank you to Anita Chopra, my dear "earthy" friend—I am certain I would have given up a million times over had it not been for your unwavering belief that I could do it. You quieted the gremlins in my head, you cheered me on, and our conversations helped get me through the tough parts. Thank you to my mom and dad, Chris and Denise Hahlen and my mother-in-law, Yvonne De Quincey, for pitching in and helping on many occasions. Thank you to my father-in-law, Ian Robertson who has read more books than anyone I have ever met; your help early in the manuscript was instrumental to start the ball rolling. Thank you to Kerry Brown whose top-notch coaching skills over the years supplied me with the tools to get the job done! Special thanks to Jenny Boychuk for your help and input. I thank all my teachers over the years that I have been so fortunate to learn from.

My deepest gratitude to my husband, Jamie, whose love and support made it all possible. Delaney, I thank you for your patience and understanding during the days that I was tucked away writing, and for letting me know when a meal or recipe was definitely not "kid-approved"! Liam and Kieran, we always joked that if your dad had not met me, he may still be feeding you corn dogs! Thank you for the joy and love you have brought to my life.

CHAPTER I

More than Nutrition

One should be mindful of what one consumes to ensure proper growth, reproduction, and development of bones, tendons, ligaments, channels, and collaterals. This will help generate the smooth flow of qi and blood, enabling one to live to a ripe age.

Maoshing Ni (1995, p.12)[1]

One winter, in my early 20s, I discovered a delightful tea called Bengal Spice®. My taste buds were head over heels for this newfound drink. This caffeine-free version of a Chai tea was brimming with cinnamon, ginger, cardamom, cloves, black pepper, and nutmeg. I started my mornings with it, drank it throughout the day, and ended with a steaming cup before bed. Oftentimes, I had as many as 10 to 12 cups per day. It had probably been about two or three months of this Bengal Spice® binging when I started to notice red outbreaks on my face. I was lucky to have had a mostly clear complexion up until this point and was perplexed as to the cause. My diet and environment were unchanged; I was using the same facial products as always, and there were no other changes that I could think of...other than the tea. I decided to cut the tea out because it was the only new addition to my life. But how could a seemingly healthy, benign, tasty cup of tea possibly be related to this breakout? The elimination of the tea did eventually clear up my skin, but I was still none the wiser—until, that is, I started my training in TCM and had my first classes in dietary therapy. The classes turned my food world upside down. I was riveted. Food could offer so much more than just feeding a hungry belly and fulfilling calories. Diet could and should

---

1   All excerpts from *The Yellow Emperor's Classic of Medicine*, translated and with commentary by Maoshing Ni, © 1995 by Maoshing Ni. Reprinted by arrangement with The Permissions Company, LLC on behalf of Shambhala Publications Inc., Boulder, Colorado (www.shambhala.com).

differ depending on the needs of an individual and their ailments. Diet could be both a preventer of disease and a slow poison. Was it a powerful medicine or a contributor to malaise? This was the beginning of a dietary paradigm shift for me.

I was able to figure out the Bengal Spice® mystery after discovering the thermal nature of food—the tea was very warming to hot in nature. The copious amounts I had been ingesting day after day had slowly caused me to "heat up" until the heat was visibly coming out of my pores in the form of acne. The tea was made wholly with spices of a *Yang* nature and had had the power to invoke a substantial change in my body.

Yin and *Yang*

The basic concepts of TCM dietary therapy are derived from the Taoist concept of *Yin* and *Yang*. *Yin* and *Yang* are opposing yet complementary forces that blend and unite to create harmony. They are interdependent— one cannot exist without the other. They transform into each other. We only know warmth because we have experienced cold. Summer changes into winter. 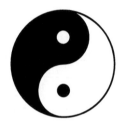 Happiness would not feel so wonderful if we had not experienced sadness. Everything in the universe can be broken down into either its *Yin* or *Yang* state.

Yin is cold, inner, night, down, soft, wet, shadow, winter, moon. *Yang* is heat, outer, day, up, hard, dry, light, summer, sun. This opposition is relative, though, as everything contains the seed of its opposite. Within *Yang* there is always a little or the beginnings of *Yin*, and within *Yin* there is always a little or the beginnings of *Yang*, which is depicted in the *Yin/Yang* symbol. Dusk and dawn are the seeds of day giving way to night and night giving way to day. *Yin* and *Yang* are relative, and something might change from *Yang* to *Yin* depending on what it is compared to—a warm spring day is *Yang* compared to a cold winter day but *Yin* when compared to a hot summer day. Children are an ever-evolving form of *Yin* into *Yang* and *Yang* into *Yin*. A sleeping baby is *Yin* in comparison to a *Yang* screaming baby. In relation to adults, children are *Yin*, but they are considered naturally *Yang* due to their energy and physical development. Their cycles of growth fluctuate between the two phases—if you've ever watched children growing, they go through a *Yin* accumulation stage where they begin to get pudgier and then suddenly sprout another inch or two, which is a growing *Yang* phase. Food therapy, likewise, in its simplest form, can categorize all food, ways of cooking, and the seasons of the year into either their *Yin* or *Yang* form. *Yin* foods have the action of cooling down the body and adding moisture, whereas *Yang* foods warm and dry the body. Some foods are *Yin* and *Yang* in perfect balance, and neither warm nor cool the body. These neutral foods are balancing and can be eaten on their own and regularly, without causing imbalances.

Thermal nature

The thermal nature of foods can be classified into cold, cooling, neutral, warming, and hot, depending on how they influence the body:

Cold	Cooling	Neutral	Warming	Hot
Salt	Fruit juices	Honey	Basil	Lamb
Seaweed	Yoghurt	Almonds	Goat's milk	Ginger
Bananas	Green peppers	Apples	Chicken	Cinnamon
Watermelon	Apples	Black beans	Walnuts	Chili peppers
Oranges	Broccoli	Carrots	Peanuts	Garlic
Lettuce	Celery	Chicken eggs	Oats	Horseradish
Shrimp	Milk	Beef	Cherries	Black pepper
Tomatoes	Cucumber	Potatoes	Prawns	Cayenne pepper

A typical Western diet for children contains a large portion of cooling and cold foods. Dairy, yoghurt, peanut butter, bananas, wheat, oranges, tomatoes, and raw vegetables are considered either cooling or cold and are common staples for children. Eating a diet abundant in cold and cooling foods can have a detrimental effect on overall digestion. This has a greater impact on children than adults due to their under-developed digestive systems. An imbalance from improper eating that might take months or years to show up in an adult can manifest in days or weeks in children. I can always tell when my daughter has had too much dairy—she will start to get a small patch of eczema along the Lung channel at her wrist, and I know it's time to cut it out for a while. Dairy creeps in more easily in the summer months in the form of ice cream—it is so hard to resist!

Refrigerating food affects its thermal nature. Food straight out of the refrigerator (or freezer) is considered cold. Cherries have a warming thermal nature, but, if served cold, they will have a cooling nature. Yoghurt has a cooling thermal nature, and if served to children directly from the fridge, this compounds the cooling effect and makes it *very cold*. Adults in the

West have become habituated to eating and drinking cold food and iced beverages and see no concern in giving the same to their children. The TCM analogy likens the stomach to a pot sitting over a fire, the fire relating to our digestive strength. This "fire" helps to break down and simmer (digest) the food. Cold and cooling food substances in excess "put out" this digestive fire and hamper digestion. Optimally, for children, eating the majority of their food within the mid-range of thermal natures (warm, cooling, and neutral), and avoiding too many foods that are in the extremes of either cold or hot, is the most beneficial for their immature organs.

How a food is prepared influences its thermal nature. For instance, raw vegetables that are cooling or cold are cooked to warm them up. Bringing cold refrigerated foods to room temperature will help to reduce their cold nature. Fruit kept stored in the fridge and brought to room temperature will "warm up" slightly without cooking. Combining cooling foods with some warming or hot food or spices will neutralize the dish—adding a pinch of cinnamon to yoghurt helps to warm it up. Lettuce is cold, but the addition of some warming herbs (rosemary, basil) in a salad dressing will balance its cooling nature. Lamb, a hot, thermal meat, is usually served with a cooling mint jelly. Sushi rolls are served with wasabi to balance out the cooling nature of the seaweed.

There are some general guidelines to figuring out what a food's thermal nature is. The longer a vegetable takes to grow, the warmer it will be for the body. Quick-growing vegetables, like lettuce, cucumber, and spinach, are cooling, whereas parsnips, pumpkin, and cabbage take months to grow and are warming. Most tropical fruit is cooling or cold and sour because it is beneficial to the people in the local environment in which it is grown—tropical climates are hot and people sweat more, so tropical fruit is eaten to clear heat, and the sour flavor produces Body Fluids. This is not the kind of fruit for a child who tends to excess mucus, that is, a phlegmy cough, nasal discharge, or postnasal drip. The spicier something is, the hotter its thermal energy; chili peppers, jalapenos, and horseradish all have hot thermal natures. Paul Pitchford, in *Healing with Whole Foods*, says that, "chemically fertilized plant foods, which are stimulated to grow quickly, are often more cooling. This includes most commercial fruits and vegetables" (2002, p.59). Eaten raw, most vegetables and fruit will be cooler than when they are cooked.

Cooking methods

Food preparation affects its thermal nature. The higher the temperature and the longer the cooking time, the more *Yang* is imparted into the dish. When food is left raw or water is used in cooking, *Yin* is imbued into the dish.

Yin → Shorter cooking times and the use of water. Eating food in its raw state. Blanching, steaming, boiling in water.

Yang → Higher heat and longer cooking times. Sautéing, baking, roasting, grilling, barbequing, slow-cooking, smoking, deep-frying, frying.

Yang methods of cooking are used in the colder seasons and *Yin* methods are used when it is warmer. Intuitively, in most cultures cooking methods tend to revolve around the seasons of the year. A warm bowl of chili sounds exactly right on a cold, snowy, winter day but not as appealing on a hot, summer day. A Canadian favorite is to barbeque meat in the summer months. Barbequing adds a lot of *Yang* to the food and would be better done in the winter months to add warmth to the body when it is cold outside!

The Five Elements

The Five Elements—Water, Wood, Fire, Earth, and Metal—are used in TCM to describe the interactions in nature, the energy flow in our bodies, how disease manifests and can be treated, our inner natures (personalities), and how the seasons flow, to name but a few. The Elements mutually "support," "generate," and "keep control" of each other when harmonious or "over-act" and "insult" each other when imbalanced. For instance, in nature, fire generates earth in the form of ash and is controlled by water (water douses a fire). An excess of water though will cause flooding and saturation of wood, creating conditions that would not be optimal for fire at all. They are used in TCM as part of the medical theory, being an extraordinarily complex methodology and treatment method. Using the Five Element connection of organs with colour, this can be a wonderfully simple way of conveying dietary balance when discussing dietary therapy with clients and how to establish it in children's diets.

The color of a food nourishes the corresponding organ. In general, the Kidneys are nourished by black foods (walnuts, seaweed, blackberries), the Liver by green foods (mung beans, celery, green leafy vegetables), the Heart by red foods (watermelon, aduki beans, beets), the Spleen by yellow foods (squash, chickpeas, sweet potatoes), and the Lungs by white foods (onions, pears, navy beans). To incorporate the five colors of food into meals helps to add diversity and ensure that all the organs are nourished. Most foods nourish more than one organ.

A fun way to include children in the process is to teach them about the five colors in food—in *real food*, that is. Smarties® do not count! "Eating the rainbow" is now promoted to children by health organizations to help incorporate many different varieties of antioxidants into the diet. Some common antioxidants in foods are:

- **Vitamin C:** found in peppers (red, green, and yellow), kiwifruit, strawberries, broccoli, and potatoes.
- **Vitamin E:** found in almonds, sunflower seeds, peanuts, sweet potatoes, and avocados.
- **Selenium:** found in Brazil nuts, fish, meat, poultry, oat bran, and eggs.
- **Carotenoids:** usually have a yellow, orange, or red color and include beta-carotene, lutein, and lycopene; found in kale, tomatoes, squash, sweet potatoes, carrots, and watermelon.
- **Flavonoids:** include anthocyanidins, flavanols, and isoflavones, and usually have a yellow, blue, black, or purple color; found in berries, especially dark berries, cherries, legumes (beans, lentils, peas, and peanuts), cocoa, olives, eggplants (also known as aubergines), and raisins.
- **Reservatrols:** found in grapes, blueberries, and peanuts.

A "color food game" that can be played at meals to encourage "rainbow eating" is to ask children to think about a "painting" they would like to create in their stomach. As they eat the different colored foods on their plates, they can be asked what it might be used for on the "canvas." Eating white rice could create a blanket of snow, peas might dot the landscape with bushes, black beans can make a sled, roasted red pepper for a sunset, and a little summer squash to color a puppy. Kids literally eat it up!

The Five Elements correspond to the seasons; winter is related to Water, spring to Wood, summer to Fire, and autumn to Metal, while the Spleen nourishes each Element during the last 18 days of each season. *The Yellow Emperor's Classic of Medicine* states, "The Spleen's placement is in the middle (center). It is the earth. In the divisions of the four seasons, the time of the spleen is the last eighteen days of each season. It does not really have a distinct season of its own" (Maoshing Ni 1995, p.116).

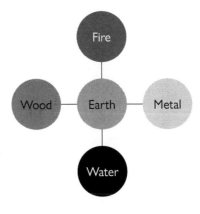

In each season, the weather and environmental conditions can affect the corresponding organ. In later chapters I discuss how to protect and nourish each organ according to the season.

Flavors

Flavor is also a distinguishing factor. The flavor attributed to each organ also nourishes and strengthens the organ when taken in moderate amounts but will do the opposite when taken in excess. Too much of a good thing is too much in this case! Salt goes to the Kidneys, sour to the Liver, bitter to the Heart, sweet to the Spleen, and pungent to the Lungs.

"In general, foods that are pungent have dispersing qualities, those that are sour have astringent qualities, sweet foods have harmonizing and decelerating qualities, bitter foods have a dispensing and drying effect, and salty foods have a softening effect," as stated in the *Neijing Suwen* (*The Yellow Emperor's Classic of Medicine*) (Maoshing Ni 1995, p.94)

Salt or naturally salty food like seaweed nourishes and moves inwards to gently nourish the Kidneys, but an excess will cause Kidney deficiency signs: weakness in the bones, increased urination, or hair loss. This corresponds with Western medicine in that an excess of salt contributes to a sodium imbalance that causes the Kidneys to have reduced function, resulting in high blood pressure.

Flavors may not exactly represent the *perceived* flavor of a given food. Herring and sardines are classified under sweet and slightly salty—salty is easy to pick out, but sweet would take a very refined palate. Most meats are classified as having a sweet thermal nature, which, in TCM dietary therapy, denotes a substance that can provide solid nourishment to the body in the form of *Qi* and blood. This is not the kind of sweet adored by children: icing, candy, or chocolate bars.

The five flavors can be used in cooking in the Five Elements' generating order, which is thought to improve overall flavor and imbue harmony into dishes. This means having at least one Element present in the dish and going in the order of generation. Wood generates Fire, Fire creates Earth, Earth holds Metal, Metal contains Water, and Water feeds Wood. This would mean starting with one of the Elements and its corresponding flavor and then following the engendering cycle when adding ingredients. You can add more than one of each Element or flavor in the sequence at a time. For instance, if it is time to add an Earth Element to the dish and you have carrots and potatoes, you may add them together and then move on to Metal. A pan that is already hot or filled with boiling hot water is considered Fire.

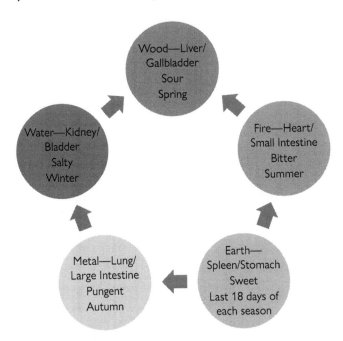

It does not matter which phase the cooking gets started in, just that it follows the engendering cycle. For instance, if making leek and potato soup, the recipe would read as follows:

Fire—Place a large saucepan on the stove. Turn to a medium heat.

Earth—Add 2 tbsp butter.

Metal—Add 1 cup of chopped onions and sauté for a few minutes.

Water—Add 1 tsp sea salt.

Wood—Add a splash of lemon juice.

Fire—Add ½ tsp thyme.

Earth—Add 2–3 chopped yellow potatoes.

Metal—Add another small pinch of thyme.

Water—Add 6 cups of chicken or vegetable stock.

Simmer the soup for 20–30 minutes.

WATER: Black/Purple foods, Kidneys/Bladder, salty, winter

WOOD: Green foods, Liver/Gallbladder, sour, spring

FIRE: Red foods, Heart/Small Intestine, bitter, summer

EARTH: Yellow/Orange foods, Spleen/Stomach, sweet, last eighteen days of each season

METAL: White foods, Lungs/Large Intestine, pungent, autumn

Direction of food

Food has the amazing ability to cause movement in the body. Individual foods can cause movement upwards, downwards, outwards, or inwards. The direction of food is an important consideration when treating illness. You would not want to use foods with an inward movement in the case of an external pathogenic factor such as wind-heat, as it may drive the factor deeper into the body.

Upwards movement: Creates movement from below the waist to the upper waist. These foods usually have a neutral or warm thermal energy, and are bitter, pungent, or sweet in flavor. These foods are important to eat in the spring as this is the season of new growth and sprouting plants. Some examples are leeks, green onions, cabbage, cinnamon, and coriander.

Downwards movement: These foods take the energy from the upper part of the body down to the lower part, and are usually of a cold, cooling, or warm thermal nature, and sour or sweet in flavor. These foods are beneficial in the autumn as the Lungs are easily affected in this season by the drier external environment, causing coughs. These foods help to reverse coughs, asthma, vomit, and acid reflux—any condition that involves a pathological reversal of energy. Apples, pears, and lemons all help to relieve a cough.

Outwards movement: These foods have the ability to push outwards to help induce sweating and expel external pathogenic factors. They are usually of a hot thermal nature and pungent or sweet in flavor. When a child is sick with a cold or flu they need foods that push outwards, like ginger, to assist in elimination of the pathogenic factor. These foods are useful to eat in the summer as they help to keep the pores open to allow for sweating.

Inwards movement: These foods create movement from the outside to the inside of the body, taking in foodstuff, especially minerals, and ensuring deep nourishment. These foods are usually of a cold thermal nature, and salty or bitter in flavor. They are beneficial in the winter as this is the season of accumulation, going inwards, hibernation, and storing up for spring, summer, and autumn. These foods are great for any bowel issues; for example, salt can pull water into the bowels, stimulating a bowel movement.

The Three Treasures, Blood and Body Fluids

These are collectively known as the Vital Substances that make up the body and mind: *Jing, Qi,* and *Shen* (Three Treasures), Blood and Body Fluids. In Chapter 3 of *The Foundations of Chinese Medicine*, Giovanni Maciocia states,

> All together, they constitute the ancient Chinese view of the body-mind. The body and mind are not seen as a mechanism (however complex) but as a vortex of energy and vital substances interacting with each other to form an organism. At the basis of all is *Qi*: all the other vital substances are but manifestations of *Qi* in varying degrees of materiality, ranging from the completely material, such as Body fluids, to the totally immaterial, such as the Mind (*Shen*). (Maciocia 1989, p.35)

The Vital Substances can all be affected and nourished or maintained by diet and digestion. The *Jing, Qi,* and *Shen* in children is said to be easily ill, easily cured. All of the Vital Substances are affected by a deficiency in the Spleen's function of acquiring *Qi* from food and drink.

Jing: Jing can be translated as Essence, and is the densest physical matter in the body. Pre-Heaven *Jing* is passed down from the mother and father and decides each child's basic root strength, creativity, fertility, and vitality. This kind of Essence is preserved by not burning the candle at both ends and by not forcing our will to do what it does not want to. Children seem to know instinctively how to preserve their *Jing*. When they are tired, they will sleep, even if it is at the dinner table. Any parent or caregiver knows that forcing them do something they do not want to do is not easy, and is often impossible. Post-Heaven *Jing* comes from the extraction of nutrients from food, fluids, and the air, which comes from the Spleen, Stomach, and

Lungs to form *Qi*. The Spleen and Stomach eventually turn food and drink into Essence, which then makes *Qi*. The Lungs create *Qi* by breathing; a lower level of energy during activity is a symptom of asthma in children. *Jing* mainly requires preserving through diet and lifestyle. A line shows up across the chin vertically when we are over-using our *Jing*—it is usually not seen on children, though it is now, unfortunately, becoming more common.

Qi: *Qi* is the life force or vitality within us. *Qi* deficiency can manifest in symptoms such as fatigue, low appetite, and loose stools. There are many forms that *Qi* takes in the body, many different hats it must wear performing different functions: Food *Qi* (*Gu Qi*), Gathering *Qi* (*Zong Qi*), True *Qi* (*Zheng Qi*), Nutritive *Qi* (*Ying Qi*), and Defensive *Qi* (*Wei Qi*). Dietary therapy is an important aspect in creating *Qi*. Spleen and Stomach *Qi* are the root of digestion and the energetic basis for producing Food *Qi*. Food *Qi* combined with air (breath) goes on to nourish all other forms of *Qi*. *Qi* is nourished by meat and fish, cooked whole grains, nuts and seeds, tempeh, tofu, and legumes. *Qi* is present in the food we eat and can be affected negatively by processing, transportation, and by an animal's living conditions and inhumane treatment. It is not hard to imagine the quality of *Qi* in an animal allowed to graze in the outdoors with access to sunshine eating its traditional diet compared to an animal raised indoors on factory farms in overcrowded spaces.

Shen: *Shen* can be translated in many ways in the English language: mind, spirit, soul, or vitality are a few examples. The *Shen* is housed or resides in the Heart and Blood Vessels and is nourished and rooted by our Blood. It is the mental, emotional, and spiritual aspect of our being and can be assessed from the sparkle and light that emanates from the eyes. The saying, "The eyes are the windows of the soul," applies beautifully here. When there is not enough Blood (Blood deficiency), we can feel ungrounded, anxious, suffer from sleep issues, and have a general lack of wellbeing. Nourishing and building the Blood is vital as it allows somewhere for the *Shen* to settle and anchor. Due to children being naturally *Yang* they can be easily stirred up, hyperactive, or have a tough time settling down; to help balance this, their *Shen* can be nourished through building the Blood (see below) and incorporating foods that calm the mind: wheat berries, wheat, celery, lavender, chamomile, valerian, passionflower, lemon balm, lemongrass, and warm milk.

Blood: Blood is a manifestation of *Qi* in a dense and material form. Blood is responsible for nourishing and moistening the body and housing the *Shen*. Blood is produced from the Food *Qi* created by the Spleen. The Spleen pushes the Food *Qi* up towards the Lungs, where it is sent to the Heart and becomes Blood. Children tend to Blood deficiency due to their immature digestive systems. This can be seen as a pale face, sleeping problems, and lack of energy. They do not make the same amount of Blood or *Qi* as adults do. Blood-nourishing foods are many of the same foods that nourish *Qi*: meat and fish, legumes, fresh vegetables, grapes, molasses, tempeh, tofu, parsley, beets, bone marrow, eggs, leafy greens, nettles, spinach, apricots, breast milk, and bone broths.

Body Fluids: In TCM there are two types of Body Fluids: Fluids (*Jin*) that are clear, light, and thin, and Liquids (*Ye*) that are turbid, heavy, and dense. The Body Fluids are derived from food and water.

Fluids (*Jin*): moisten skin and muscles and manifest as sweat, tears, saliva, and mucus; a component in Blood to prevent stasis.

Liquids (*Ye*): moisten the joints, spine, brain, and bone marrow, and lubricate the orifices of the ears, eyes, nose, and mouth.

Fluids and Liquids are both *Yin* substances in the body, and symptoms are seen in the form of dryness (dry skin, constipation, thirst) or in the accumulation of phlegm fluids. To moisten dryness and lubricate the body, *Yin*-nourishing foods that create Body Fluids are indicated: apples, pears, apricots, sweet potatoes, yams, spinach, tofu, coconut milk, oysters, and tomatoes. When there is an excess of phlegm fluids, nourishing the Spleen will aide in transforming and transporting fluids; the following foods help to rid the body of excess moisture: alfalfa, barley, asparagus, celery, corn silk, Job's tears, peas, rice, and water chestnuts.

CHAPTER 2

The Immature Spleen Craves Sweetness

The function of the spleen is to transform and transport the essence of food and fluids of the stomach. The symbology of the earth is to nourish all things in nature. It is all-encompassing. It is responsible for nourishing every single part of the body.

Maoshing Ni (1995, p.12)

The Spleen and Stomach (Middle Burner) hold a position of the highest order in TCM. They are the main organs responsible for the creation of postnatal Essence (*Jing*) (acquired constitution), which begins to be produced immediately after birth with the first suckles of milk entering the baby's stomach, and their first cries bringing air deep into their lungs. This is the beginning of the process whereby *Qi* and Blood are created to nourish all the other organs and to create the Body Fluids (*Jin/Ye*) used for nourishing and moistening the skin, muscles, joints, spine, brain, bone marrow, and all the orifices (eyes, ears, nose, and mouth). Postnatal Essence is dependent on lifestyle factors for its replenishment and is a major contributor to the energy and health of an individual child: healthy food and drink, adequate sleep, a balance between work and rest, and a nurturing environment are all positive influences.

In the womb, babies are nourished by prenatal Essence (congenital constitution). Prenatal Essence is inherited from both the mother and father at conception and is also dependent on nourishment from the mother during gestation. Prenatal Essence is decided at birth and can be *protected* by striving for balance in life and by not burning the candle at both ends, but cannot be replenished daily, as is the case with postnatal Essence. Prenatal Essence, at birth, is set for life: the words of my daughter's preschool teacher

29

ring true in regard to our congenital constitution, "You get what you get, and you don't get upset." Some must work harder at producing postnatal Essence as their prenatal Essence reserve is less than others. TCM makes it clear that although someone is born with a strong congenital constitution, this doesn't warrant a free ride; squandered and left neglected, prenatal Essence can dwindle, causing ensuing impairment. Children's Spleens are inherently weak until around the age of seven. Because the Spleen has such a vital role to play in the production of postnatal Essence, dietary therapies aimed at supporting and strengthening this important organ in children are paramount. Positively nourishing their postnatal Essence is insurance towards health and vitality throughout life. To neglect the Spleen and diet in children is akin to neglecting the soil, sun, and water when planting a seedling; the foundation and its sustenance are crucial to its maturation.

A Harvard report, titled *The Foundations of Lifelong Health Are Built in Early Childhood*, from the Center on the Developing Child (2010, p.4), identifies three domains for the *foundations of health in the early years that can exert either a positive or negative influence on physical and mental wellbeing: a stable and responsive environment of relationships* (consistent, nurturing and protective interactions with adults), *safe and supportive physical, chemical and built environments*, and (most importantly!) *sound and appropriate nutrition*—health-promoting food intake and eating habits, beginning with the mother's pre-conception nutritional status.

Food *Qi*

The Spleen is one of the five *Zang* organs in the body. *Zang* is a TCM term for the viscera, which includes the Kidney, Liver, Heart, Spleen, and Lungs, all of which are *Yin* organs that store *Qi* and Blood. Its paired organ, the Stomach, is one of the six *Fu* organs. *Fu* is a TCM term for the *Yang* organs, which include the Bladder, Gallbladder, Triple Burner, Small Intestine, Stomach, and Large Intestine. The Spleen and Stomach are the *Yin* and *Yang* pair of the Earth element. The Earth produces plants and supplies water, which is essential to its inhabitants' survival. The Earth cannot thrive with excess water or flooding. The Spleen is the same—dampness encumbers its functions. The Earth also suffers without enough water (dryness), which results in cracking and the discouragement of most plant, flower, and tree growth. Likewise, the Stomach does not like dryness and likes to stay moist.

The Spleen and Stomach work together to ensure the transformation and transportation of food and drink. Food and drink are initially broken down in the Stomach; the Stomach decides what to send to the Spleen for further transformation and the rest is sent down to the Small Intestine for further separation and absorption. The Spleen is responsible for taking the food that has been churned in the Stomach and turning it into Food *Qi* (*Gu Qi*), which is a process of extracting the energy from foodstuff. The Spleen then lifts this Food *Qi* up to the chest where it goes to the Lungs. In the Lungs, Food *Qi* combines with Clear *Qi*, which comes from the air we breathe, to form Gathering *Qi* (*Zong Qi*). Gathering *Qi* is an even more refined form of *Qi*, which is further transformed in the Lungs into True *Qi* (*Zheng Qi*). True *Qi* has two forms: Nutritive *Qi* (*Ying Qi*), which ends up circulating in the body and through the channels (aka, meridians) and to all the organs in the form of nourishment, and Defensive *Qi* (*Wei Qi*), which flows along the exterior of the body, its main function to protect against exterior pathogenic factors, such as Wind, Cold, Heat, and Damp. The strength of Defensive *Qi* decides our immune system; this highlights the connection of proper diet to our immunity. Food *Qi* sent from the Spleen also goes to the Heart where it becomes Blood. This whole process relies heavily on the Stomach's ability to transform food and the Spleen's ability to *lift* Food *Qi* upwards. It is also reliant on the quality of food and drink. *Food is the foundation of all Qi and Blood in the body.*

Bubbling cauldron

In TCM, the Stomach is likened to a pot sitting above a source of heat that comes from the Spleen (Spleen *Yang*) to keep the pot simmering. The simmering pot is essentially the churning and chemical breakdown of food that occurs in the Stomach. The Spleen *Yang* is kept warm by the life gate fire (Ming Men Fire). As the food cooks in the pot, the pure and the turbid are separated. The Spleen takes the pure food essences from the Stomach, and the transformation and transportation process (Spleen *Qi*) creates *Qi* and Blood. The Stomach likes to be moist, or the pot may dry out or burn, whereas the Spleen likes to stay dry so as not to put the heat source out. If the Spleen energy is insufficient, food will not be broken down properly and it will be more difficult for the body to obtain nutrients. This will also affect its ability to transform and transport fluids, leading to a build-up of dampness, which will further hamper the Spleen's ability due to the water or dampness impeding the digestive fire. Alternatively, if there is too much fire, food burns away too quickly and there can be frequent hunger, constipation, or a strong desire for cold drinks.

The immature Spleen

The digestive system takes about seven years from birth to fully develop, and it is very immature in the first two years of life. It is during this time when "food accumulation disorders" can arise, especially in infants, where food collects (backs up) in the stomach and intestines. The *Zhong Yi Er Ke Xue* (*The Study of Chinese Medicine Pediatrics*) says, "Children's transportation and transformation function is not fortified and complete; therefore, they are easily damaged by food" (quoted in Flaws 1996). Therefore, children are prone to digestive disorders: stomach ache, constipation, diarrhea, nausea, low appetite, colic, and bloating are all common childhood ailments. If the Spleen is not transforming and transporting fluids properly, they will accumulate and go to the Lungs in the form of excess mucus and phlegm, causing problems such as wheezing, asthma, allergies, a cough, and a runny nose. Children need protection from the outside world by being shown what's safe and what isn't, getting bundled up to protect them from the cold, and slathering sunscreen on them when it's a hot day; in the same way, they require digestive protection and supplementation.

Signs of a balanced Spleen and Stomach:

- Regular daily bowel movements with no undigested food.
- Normal appetite (this can fluctuate in children depending on growth cycles).
- Lots of energy.

Signs of Spleen and Stomach deficiency:

- Low appetite.
- Nausea.
- Stomach aches.
- Loose stools with undigested food or diarrhea.
- Constipation.
- Bloating.
- Eczema.
- Runny nose.
- Frequent colds.
- Allergies (food, environmental).
- Blue coloring between the eyes at the bridge of the nose; this can be due to an inability to digest lactose or may be a sign of excess sugar in the diet. It can also be a result of the mother eating excess sugar during pregnancy or while breastfeeding.

Pernicious influences affecting the Spleen
Dairy

Dairy is difficult to digest and has a cool thermal nature. It is often served directly from the refrigerator, increasing its cold thermal nature. A little dairy for children is not a problem as it is supplementing to the Spleen in small amounts, nourishes *Qi* and Blood, and is indicated for weakness and exhaustion. However, too much dairy in the diet will weaken the Spleen and Stomach, and can lead to dampness and phlegm accumulation. Fermented dairy, such as yoghurt, kefir, certain cheeses, and cream cheese are better tolerated as some contain probiotics and the milk has already been partially digested by the bacteria. Warming up the milk, adding a pinch of ginger or turmeric, and not serving milk with other foods are all ways to decrease its dampening effects.

It is always important to assess dairy intake in infants and children as it can have a substantial effect on their overall health and the functioning of their Middle Burner. Ghee is an alternative to butter; it has minimal lactose and casein. Both butter and ghee contain high amounts of butyrate acid, a saturated short-chain fatty acid; high levels of butyrate in the gut has been used as an indicator of a healthy microbiome (Pryde *et al.* 2002). Mother's milk is far superior to cow dairy, and if possible, recommended to be the only source of milk for the first six months of life. If breastfeeding is not an option, goat milk formulas are preferable as they are easier to digest and are less damp-forming.

Too much raw food

Most raw vegetables and fruit are cooling. An excess of raw food in the diet will weaken the Spleen. Cooking food helps its digestibility and is warming. Cooking also softens the plants' cell walls, releasing more of the nutrients that are bound to the wall itself. Some cooked vegetables also supply more antioxidants, such as beta-carotene, lutein, and lycopene. As you will learn in the chapters ahead, the amount of raw food you consume should ebb and flow with the seasons. This makes sense when you look at what grows locally in each season. For example, it is difficult to eat the raw root vegetables that are available in winter compared to the lettuce leaves and tomatoes of summer. The body also requires cooling in the summer and warming in the winter to achieve balance and to stay healthy.

Chilled, frozen, or iced foods

Our Western culture loves cold food and drink! It can feel incredibly refreshing to pop some ice into our water on a hot day—we feel like we are cooling ourselves down. However, our bodies have to *warm up* to balance the cold that consumes *Yang Qi*. In Eastern cultures, it is well known that cold food and drink is not healthy. In fact, eventually our bodies do not even feel the effects of ingesting food or drinks that are ice-cold or refrigerator-cold unless we give ourselves a break from them. "Brain freeze" (the scientific term is sphenopalatine ganglioneuralgia), that unpleasant phenomenon I am sure we have all experienced at one point or another, is the body's way of telling us that we've ingested something cold too quickly. It is too bad the Spleen doesn't have a strong regulator like brain freeze to alarm us any time there is chilled food or drink in the system. It would be a lot easier to notice the ill effects immediately!

Chilled foods include anything that comes right out of the fridge or freezer and goes straight into the mouth and belly. TCM has always stated that the best temperature to ingest food and drink at is warm or room temperature. The cold does to the inside of the body what it does to the outside: it contracts tissue and prevents blood flow. This is the opposite of how we want digestion to function; we want enzymes flowing and the stomach muscles to be relaxed. Occasional cold food, like ice cream in the summer, will not have long-term adverse effects on the Middle Burner in children—it is the daily ice cubes in drinks, cold yoghurt, or smoothies made with frozen berries that will have a negative impact over time.

Damp-forming foods

These are foods that eventually weaken the Spleen and thus engender dampness. One of my clients, during her treatment with me, was complaining about how her young boys' noses were always running, even though they were not sick. I inquired about their diets. Mandarin oranges were a regular snack in their household, sometimes up to three or four a day per child! I suggested trying to eliminate the mandarins for a few weeks to find out if this could be the contributing factor. When I next saw my client, she told me that the boys' runny noses had finally cleared. Children's bodies are amazing and most often able to recover quickly! In TCM we say the Earth element (Spleen and Stomach) creates dampness and the Metal element (Lungs and Large Intestine) stores it. Therefore, dampness from the Spleen can instantly affect the Lungs, causing coughing or wheezing, as well as the Large Intestine, which presents with rumbling and loose stools.

Some common damp-forming foods include:

- Excess sugar and sweets.
- Fruit juice (excess sweetness).
- Consuming chilled, frozen, or iced food or drink regularly.
- Refined starch and white flour.
- Excess raw fruits (especially tropical fruit, including bananas) and vegetables.
- Excess nuts (especially peanut butter).
- Excess dairy.
- Excess mushrooms.
- Excess of fatty, greasy, and fried foods.
- Smoothies (made with frozen berries or raw greens).

Sugar

In adults, one of the determining indicators of a Spleen deficiency is a craving for sweets. Children have this natural craving because of their immature and inherently weak Spleen and Stomach system. While the Spleen requires the sweet taste to function well, we know that too much of a good thing can create an opposite (and unwanted) effect. Chinese dietary therapy recommends naturally sweet food to satisfy this craving. Starchy vegetables and the natural sweetness in oats and grains are traditionally favored when we talk about the addition of a "sweet" flavor that nourishes the Spleen.

The longer parents can keep sugar out of a child's diet, the better. Besides, when children are young, they do not know what they are missing! Why introduce sugar early on when there is simply no reason to? This is where Western societal conditioning could use a reset. So often, "treats" (i.e., sweets) are used as a reward, associated with a fun occasion, or are even used as a manipulative tool. As a result, it then becomes difficult for children to appreciate naturally sweet flavors, as they have become desensitized from consuming so much refined white sugar. It is also more difficult to introduce new foods or flavors once they are habituated to such high levels of sweetness. Consequently, once children are desensitized to the natural sweetness of foods, it takes time to get them back to a place where food is appreciated on its own (without the addition of sugar or other sweeteners).

I hope to see our Western society strive to embrace and create mindfulness around our children's sugar intake. As a parent, I often feel like an outsider in this regard. I see refined white sugar show up more and more in children's everyday lives in the form of cupcakes, donuts, and cookies, which are brought to school for every child's birthday (keep in mind that this could be up to 25 times in a school year, which doesn't even include birthday parties!), popsicles, or other sugary frozen treats given out for fun days at school, candy or chocolate given out on Valentine's Day, and all the other myriad ways "treats" are distributed. Each season brings a plethora of seasonal or holiday-themed chocolate and candy in stores. It is interesting to witness this seasonal flow of offerings once you become aware of it! Christmas, Valentine's Day, Easter, Mother's Day, Halloween... Round and round the candy carousel goes! I have found it becomes more difficult to steer clear of sugar as children get older and start to attend school, birthday parties, go off trick or treating, or attend the multitude of other events where some form of sugar seems to have somehow become the focus.

Limiting or completely avoiding refined white sugar, white refined flours, and sweetened beverages for as long as possible is one of the best ways to support a child's Spleen function. Parents need to know how to read labels and identify the kind and the amount of sugar in processed foods. It is well known that sugar hides in the food supply in the form of tomato sauces, salad dressings, granola bars, etc., and the best way to avoid hidden sugar is to buy unprocessed foods and to cook as much possible from scratch. This is not always an easy endeavor for busy families, but there are companies striving to limit or eliminate sugar in their products.

Practitioner tip:
Create a list of locally made or commercially produced products that are easily found in your region that have little or no sugar.

There are many different variations of sugar that show up in our food (*especially* children's foods and snacks)—up to 300 different names to date![1]

Here are the more common ways sugar is labeled:

- Sugar or sucrose: chemically processed and highly refined.
- Organic cane sugar or sweetener: *just* as processed as white refined

---

1   If you are interested in learning more, a great online resource can be found at www. Robertlustig.com—Robert H. Lustig MD, MSL, Professor Emeritus of Pediatrics, Division of Endocrinology at the University of California, San Francisco, specializes in the field of neuroendocrinology, with an emphasis on the regulation of energy balance by the central nervous system. His research and clinical practice focus on childhood obesity and diabetes.

sugar, but in this case the sugar cane is grown using organic farming and processing methods and has not been genetically modified (non-GMO).

- Fructose: 100 percent metabolized by the Liver and not used for cellular energy. Robert H. Lustig has called it "alcohol without the buzz." Research has shown it to be the cause of metabolic syndrome, obesity, and type 2 diabetes.
- High-fructose corn syrup: similar in effect as fructose, but with more fructose than sugar. In Canada this is labeled as glucose-fructose.
- Coconut sugar: made from the sap of the coconut tree, which is extracted, boiled, and then dehydrated. It is high in fructose, which, as we know, goes directly to the Liver for processing.
- Agave nectar: often thought of as a "healthier" sweetener. However, because it is made by treating agave sugars with heat and enzymes, any beneficial minerals are destroyed, and the end product is a highly refined, unhealthy syrup. Agave nectar is high in fructose—as high as 55 to 97 percent—which makes it an even unhealthier alternative to high-fructose corn syrup.
- Brown sugar: refined white sugar that has had molasses added for color and flavor, or it can also be a slightly less-refined sugar that is allowed to retain some of its natural flavor and natural brown color.
- Dextrose: a simple sugar derived from corn.
- Unrefined raw cane sugar: GMO-free, grown without synthetic pesticides and fertilizers, and uses organic farming and processing methods. It is unrefined and still contains some of the molasses and moisture from the plant.

For home baking and use as a sweetener, I recommend the following types of sweeteners:

- Maple syrup: high in antioxidants, this makes a good baking substitute for refined sugars.
- Blackstrap molasses: low sugar content, high in iron, and benefits anemia.
- Barley malt syrup: unrefined liquid sweetener made from soaked and sprouted barley. On the sweetness scale, fructose is a 10, while barley malt syrup is a 2. A great way to add subtle sweetness.
- Honey: should be used sparingly—it is not safe to give to infants under one year of age due to bacterial spores that can cause infant botulism, a rare, but potentially life-threatening, disease. Honey is

much sweeter than white sugar and raises blood sugar levels quickly. It does have some healing properties, though; it is antibacterial, antifungal, a good source of antioxidants, and a prebiotic. It strengthens the Spleen and Stomach and is neutral in temperature. A little honey used medicinally or occasionally is fine, but because of its high level of sweetness, too much will weaken the Spleen.

- Stevia: native to South America. The sweetening power of this plant is several hundred times stronger than white sugar! Look for the green or brown extracts or powders, but avoid white or clear extracts, which have been highly refined. This sweetener has no effect on blood sugar or insulin response.

The emotional Spleen

A child's Spleen is also nourished through their connection to Earth. Mother Earth is the figure that represents sustenance, nourishment, love for all, and home for people, plants, and animals. For children, this is literally their motherly figure, whoever that may be. The emotional Spleen is nurtured when the child feels grounded, feels a sense of security, and has a place to call home. Touch also nourishes the Spleen. We know that babies who are not held, nuzzled, and cuddled can stop growing—and, if the absence goes on for long enough, they can die. The importance of physical touch is just as important for survival and growth as necessities like food and water. Dr Frederick Leboyer, a French obstetrician and author, said, "Being touched and caressed, being massaged, is food for the infant. Food as necessary as minerals, vitamins, and proteins" (1999, p.20).

Daverick Leggett, author of *Recipes for Self-Healing*, writes

Archetypally the Spleen is related to the mother. In the process of growing up the needs that are initially provided for by the mother are increasingly provided for by the growing child itself. Eventually a person develops an "internal mother," an ability to find comfort and nourishment from within. At this point in development the Spleen energy can be said to be mature. (1999, p.45)

Nourishing the Middle Burner

Nourishing the Spleen and Stomach in children can prevent many unnecessary ailments and seeks to reduce illness severity and frequency. As more is discovered about the gut microbiome and its connection to health, the more it becomes apparent that what we eat truly impacts our health for better or worse, and the younger years are formative in this regard. Many of the common childhood ailments discussed in Chapter 9 refer to this part of the book for treatment, as a weak Spleen is a common etiology occurring in children.

Beneficial foods for the Spleen

You might remember certain foods and home-cooked meals you had when you were growing up, which you now crave, foods or meals that bring back good memories when you eat them. For me, it is a cheese fondue or cave-aged Gruyère cheese (I come from a Swiss heritage). A pile of cubed bread sitting beside a pot of simmering, bubbling cheese will always fill my bucket, and cave-aged Gruyère cheese sends off fireworks in my mouth. This kind of nostalgic meal elicits a totally different internal satisfaction and nourishes our Spleen over and above what would normally be considered healthy, even in TCM terms. Only a small amount of this food is required and will satisfy the craving and create *Qi*. The more enjoyment there is towards what is eaten, the more *Qi* is created. Joy is the emotion connected to the Heart, and the Heart (Fire) feeds and nurtures the Spleen (Earth). I feel it is important to mention this first, as I believe mealtime is sacred and that the atmosphere surrounding mealtimes is equally as important as the food itself!

Though I will list the foods known in TCM to be nourishing to the Spleen and Stomach, it is vital to know that there is simply more to nourishing ourselves than just nutrients. My wonderful teacher, Lillian Bridges—the world's leading authority on face reading and diagnosis in TCM—teaches that one way of deeply nurturing the Spleen is with meals that feel as if we are "feeding our souls." These might be foods or meals from childhood, or even foods or meals that come from our DNA, our ancestry. For example, someone with Scandinavian roots might crave fatty fish, whereas someone with Middle Eastern roots might crave falafels. These craved foods will supply the body with more energy than regular meals because they make the Spleen *so happy*. A plate of poutine (French fries, cheese curds and brown gravy), which I do not think anyone would qualify as being "healthy," could be a potential *Qi* maker if it generates these feelings. Only a small amount of this craved food is needed to satisfy the craving and hunger; this is not the same, however, as when a child binges on their Halloween candy and ends up with a sugar rush followed by the all too familiar sugar crash symptoms:

grumpy, whiny, tired, sick, or dizzy. Instead, the kind of deep nourishment given by these certain foods and meals that a child may ask for specifically will engender a satiated, content, and fulfilled feeling. As practitioners who recommend dietary therapy for children, we must also keep in mind that enjoyment of food is paramount.

For the immature Spleen to be nurtured by diet, foods must be easily digestible, cooked, and have natural sweetness. Children best enjoy food that is slightly bland. Too much spice or flavoring can be too intense and overwhelming for their undeveloped taste buds, whereas the sweet taste nourishes and relaxes the Spleen. Root vegetables, whole grains, beans, rice, and proteins are the foods that are considered most beneficial for the Spleen. From an evolutionary standpoint, sweet (and salty) flavors are biologically preferred over other flavors, such as bitterness. This is because sweet foods are higher in calories and were not previously found in abundance. Bitterness could also potentially signal a poisonous food and something to stay away from.

Research by Julie Mennella shows that within hours of birth, children exhibit a strong preference for sweet tastes, which eventually declines when they reach mid-adolescence and coincides with cessation of growth (Mennella and Bobowski 2015). Their taste buds prefer concentrated sweets. Dr Mennella's research found that an adult's most preferred level of sucrose is equivalent to 0.3 molar, which is about what a Coca-Cola® tastes like. A child's preferred level is double, at 0.6 molar. This is biologically helpful because it guides them to prefer breast milk, which is naturally sweet, and during periods of heightened growth they become more attracted to foods like fruit and honey, which contain more calories to sustain this development. Plus, sugar is a natural analgesic, which helps to mitigate pain while growing. From an evolutionary standpoint, these are all good reasons to favor sweet foods.

Knowing that children have this strong preference for sweetness, it is easy to see how vulnerable they are to today's food environments of sugar-laden snacks and desserts. Children cannot easily say "no" when offered candy because they are not biologically wired to do so.

The more *naturally* sweet foods we offer to children, the less hungry they will be for empty calories. It is no coincidence that our bodies need sweetness to nourish the Spleen, which is the organ responsible for transforming and transporting food into usable nutrients for the body, or that sweetness is the flavor that naturally lures us towards foods that are higher in calories, sustain energy levels, and assist with growth.

The longer a food is cooked, the easier it becomes to digest, and the more nourishing it is for the Spleen. Congee is used for this reason in China and kitchari in India—slow-cooked, easy to digest meals of rice, suitable for helping recovery when ill. For children these are great in-between meals when they may have had a run of sweets, dairy, and greasy foods and require a system reset.

VEGETABLES

All root vegetables and squash varieties are especially nourishing for the Spleen. Vegetables with a yellow or orange color have an affinity for the Spleen and Stomach.

- Beets
- Cabbage
- Carrots
- Cauliflower
- Corn
- Onions
- Parsnips
- Potatoes
- Sweet potatoes
- Red and yellow peppers
- Rutabaga (swede)
- Turnips
- Vegetable broth soups
- Winter squash (pumpkin, acorn, spaghetti, butternut, delicata, kabocha, etc.)
- Yams.

FRUITS

Seasonal and local fruit are the best options for nourishing and harmonizing. An excess of fruit will weaken the Spleen. Juicing fruit increases their cooling properties.

- Apples
- Blueberries
- Cantaloupe
- Cherries
- Dates
- Figs
- Grapes
- Raisins
- Strawberries.

LEGUMES AND PULSES

These are all superfoods; they are high in fiber and provide protein, as well as being significant sources of vitamins and minerals.

- Chickpeas
- Lentils (yellow, orange, green, brown, and black)
- Peas
- Kidney beans
- Black beans
- Pinto beans
- White beans
- Adzuki beans
- Fava beans
- Green beans
- Snow peas
- Lima beans

- Split peas
- Soybeans (yellow and black).

GRAINS

Grains should make up the bulk of the diet. They are very nourishing to the Spleen and Stomach and are usually well received by children. Grains can be soaked before cooking to improve digestibility.

- Amaranth
- Barley
- Buckwheat
- Corn
- Job's tears
- Rice
- Rye
- Sweet rice
- Millet
- Oats
- Spelt.

MEAT AND FISH

Small amounts of meat and fish nourish the Spleen.

- Chicken
- Beef
- Duck
- Herring
- Mackerel
- Goat
- Salmon
- Trout
- Tuna
- Halibut
- Turkey
- Lamb
- Venison, moose, elk
- Bone broths.

NUTS AND SEEDS

Small amounts of nuts nourish the Spleen. Lightly roasting the nuts before eating will make them easier to digest. Soaking the nuts before blending or cooking with them will improve their flavor and will also aid with digestibility.

- Almonds
- Brazil nuts
- Cashews
- Coconut
- Chestnuts
- Hazelnuts
- Pistachios
- Peanuts
- Pumpkin seeds
- Sunflower seeds.

SPICES

- Aniseed
- Black pepper
- Caraway seeds
- Cardamom
- Coriander
- Cumin
- Dill seeds
- Fennel
- Licorice

- Ginger
- Marjoram
- Nutmeg
- Oregano
- Rosemary
- Star anise
- Thyme
- Turmeric.

SWEETENERS

A small amount of natural sweetener nourishes the Spleen.

- Dates
- Molasses
- Barley malt
- Maple syrup
- Honey.

DAIRY

Minimal amounts; an excess of dairy in the diet will engender dampness.

- Butter
- Ghee.

Other considerations for the Spleen
Eat at regular times each day

The saying in TCM is "the Spleen likes regularity," which means eating meals at roughly the same time every day is the most beneficial for digestion. These days, there seems to be a trend towards allowing children to graze all day on snacks. A lot of the processed snacks are wheat- and/or sugar-based and cause a spike in blood sugar, which is then quickly followed with a drop in blood sugar. This creates a cycle of constant hunger. Then, come lunch or dinner, their little bellies are too full to eat a proper meal. It is important that the stomach has a chance to empty before the next meal. We should consider that, because children's stomachs are smaller than ours, they *will* need more frequent, smaller meals. So, how to balance the need for more frequent meals while discouraging over-snacking?

First, we recommend that children eat their breakfast or lunch in two sittings, if need be. Sometimes 10 minutes later they are ready for a little more food. The same goes for dinner. Main meals will contain higher amounts of fat and protein, which should reduce the requests and need for as many snacks between meals—7–9am is when the *Qi* enters the Stomach in the organ body clock, and is the optimal time for breakfast.

Chew food well

Digestion begins in the mouth, and children are usually great at chewing and taking their time with meals. When a child presents with a digestive issue, it will be important to rule out any issues surrounding how they chew their food.

Stress-free mealtimes

A relaxed environment, free from the stresses of the day, will allow the digestive system to relax. This also means focusing on the meal and not watching television, playing video games, or even reading. The stress response is meant to inhibit digestion to allow the body to prepare for fight or flight.

CHAPTER 3

Taijiao: The Importance of Our Time in the Womb

Gardeners know that you must nourish the soil if you want healthy plants. You must water the plants adequately, especially when seeds are germinating and sprouting, and they should be planted in a nutrient-rich soil. Why should nutrition matter less in the creation of young humans than it does in young plants? I'm sure that it doesn't.

Gaskin (2003, p.215)

Generally, when someone has gone through five months of pregnancy, the child in the womb can often make small indications of movement, as if to announce itself to its mother, and the mother thereupon responds by stroking [her belly], connecting via her will. Their spirits communicate back and forth, like a radio transmitting without pause until the completion to nine months. Thereupon, coming into the world with a cry, the pearl in the middle of one's belly will emerge like a precious jewel in the palm of one's hand.

Richardson (2011, p.3)

What if there was a possibility to increase the wellbeing of the future world population? A universal remedy of sorts meant to decrease the rates of obesity, heart disease, diabetes, and many other chronic diseases? What if you could impart health benefits that could trickle down to subsequent generations? A way for children to get a head start in life, physically and mentally, that could extend into adulthood? This way might lie in the placenta during the 280 days of gestation.

We are blessed to live in a time where we have realized the dangers that alcohol, smoking, certain foods, and pharmaceuticals have on the fetus so

45

as not repeat them, and are very careful of what is prescribed to pregnant women. It is now known that these substances have the potential to cause immediate harm to the fetus and so are best avoided. This immediate harm is easier to determine earlier on in a child's life, but the long-term health outcomes—mental health, chronic disease, and how we handle stress—could these health outcomes also have their roots in the womb?

Chinese culture, from the time of the Han dynasty, has always thought of pregnancy as the time when the fetus first begins its education and starts to learn about the world outside its warm, safe womb cocoon (Li 2009). Pregnancy is, most often, a joyful, exciting time for women, a true miracle of life. Coupled with this excitement there can also be worry and fear about doing or not doing or eating or not eating something that might harm the fetus. Warnings on labels, "Not for pregnant or nursing women," and the lists of foods and scents and activities to avoid can be overwhelming. With these in mind, the information given here is meant to uplift women and to offer recommendations that are based on TCM theory and also modern findings. Our medicine has so much to offer pregnant women—dietary and lifestyle advice, acupuncture, herbal remedies, nonpharmaceutical pain relief, Qi Gong, meditation, and more. Instead of medicalizing pregnancy, we can instead miraculize it.

Sun Simiao, famously known as the "King of Medicinals," lived in China from around 581–682. His philosophy was that the treatment of women and children should be of the utmost importance, and that by taking care of women and children, the foundations of a healthy family would be supported, and, in turn, subsequent generations. He placed the treatment of women at the beginning of his book, *Bei Ji Qian Jin Yao Fang* (*Prescriptions Worth a Thousand in Gold for Every Emergency*), followed by the treatment of children. As more is researched and understood about pregnancy and fetal development, the more it makes sense to regard the care of woman (and especially pregnant women) and children as paramount, since the time spent in the womb seems to have lifelong implications. The months in utero seem to be a crucial aspect in determining someone's health trajectory. Sun Simiao was ahead of his time to have considered this 1400 years ago.

Taijiao and the fetal origins hypothesis

Much of our modern-day education regarding pregnancy involves the care and attention required post-partum. Many soon-to-be parents will attend classes that prepare them for the upcoming labor, how to care for their newborn baby, breastfeeding information, swaddling instructions, how often to feed, when to introduce solids, etc., but there is very little or no talk at all about the importance of the time in the womb. Taijiao translates as "fetal education." Its use in TCM dates back well over 2000 years. The underpinnings of Taijiao have always taught and believed that what the mother ingests—whether it is what's going into her body or what she reads and listens to and feels in her spirit—will affect the fetus in either a positive or negative way.

The "Barker hypothesis," now also known as the "fetal origins hypothesis," was first brought to light (in our Western medical system) by epidemiologist and British physician, David J. Barker, who found a connection between low birth weight and future rates of heart disease and metabolic disorders (Barker and Martyn 1992). It offered an explanation as to why such a high number of adult males who fell into low-risk categories for plasma lipid concentrations, blood pressure, smoking, and pre-existing symptoms for coronary heart disease were dying of coronary heart disease (Rose 1985). Barker wrote that the "womb may be more important than the home" (1990, p.1111). Subsequent studies have confirmed the link between low birth weight leading to obesity, diabetes, and cardiovascular disease later in life (Burton, Fowden, and Thornburg 2016; Jornayvaz *et al.* 2016). This theory is now a commonly accepted fact. The gestation period has a major and significant influence in laying down our foundations of health in life. On the flip side, this research also confirms that certain factors, such as smoking, excess stress, or lack of nutrients can have deleterious effects.

Practices taught in Taijiao were rooted in principles observed long before the time of the Barker hypothesis. Taijiao teaches that the wellbeing of the pregnant mother should be held in utmost importance as the health of future generations lies within.

Parts of the Taijiao principles are related to what is optimal for the mother to eat—not only ensuring her health is protected, but also the health of her fetus. Dietary therapy for children can start right when there is a positive pregnancy test! Moreover, in TCM it is recommended that women spend a minimum of three to six months before trying to conceive getting the "soil ready for implantation"; enriching the uterine lining, attuning the cycle, and nourishing the body in preparation for the fertilized egg. Three to six months is about the time required for a follicle to fully mature before potentially being released during ovulation. This is done to ensure a strong, healthy pregnancy, and to reduce the chance of miscarriage. A 2018 article in the science journal *The Lancet* from Stephenson *et al.* (2018, p.1830) found that "a woman who is healthy at the time of conception is more likely to have successful pregnancy and a healthy child." They called for a heightened awareness of preconception health, particularly regarding diet and nutrition. A few great TCM resources that lay out beneficial methods for the body pre-conception and to optimize fertility can be found in Dr Randine Lewis, *The Infertility Cure*, Aimee E. Raupp, *Yes, You Can Get Pregnant*, and Daoshing Ni, *The Tao of Fertility*.

Pregnancy can be a powerfully motivating force in a woman's life to make optimal lifestyle and dietary changes, when the health of the body and reproductive system affects a little being other than themselves. As practitioners, we have a wonderful opportunity to really help our pregnant women feel better, both mentally and physically. We have the opportunity to create a dialogue around the positive impact they can have on their future child while in utero; this is the true art of preventative medicine that is the cornerstone of TCM.

At the same time, we must also acknowledge that this awareness can induce worry and anxiety. Societal pressures on pregnant women can be intense; in our modern lives it is not always easy to follow the recommendations to remain stress-free and adhere to a nutritional plan. This is not the objective. The objective here is "knowledge is power," and that we should all do the best we can with what we have in our lives at that very moment.

The history of Taijiao

One of the earliest known texts to emerge on the subject of Taijiao was excavated from Mawangdui's ("King Ma's Mound") archeological site in Hunan province, China, in the early 1970s. These manuscripts were buried in 168 BCE, and so dated before then. The *Taichanshu* (*Book of Gestation and Birth*) was one of the manuscripts found inside the tomb along with many other relics, including the *Yijing* (*Classic of Changes*) and the *Tao Te Jing* (*The Classic of the Way and Virtue*). "This early silk manuscript contains a month-by-month account of the fetal developmental characteristics for a particular month along with diet and behavioral prescriptions for the expectant mother; the understanding of embryology was amazingly advanced at this time" (Wilms and Betts n.d.).

In the Han dynasty (206 BCE–220 CE), Taijiao was greatly stressed. Scholar, Liu Xiang, advocated for fetal education to sculpt the moral characteristics of the child at the earliest phase—in utero. Prescriptions were written for what women should see, hear, eat, and say, and how to conduct themselves in a polite and proper manner. Liu Xiang said that if a woman was affected by good things, her child would be good, if she was affected by bad things, the child would be bad (Kinney n.d.). She should not allow evil sights or sounds in her life, lest they influence the fetus negatively.

Sun Simiao also wrote about fetal education in an essay included in his book, *Bei Ji Qian Jin Yao Fang* (*Prescriptions Worth a Thousand in Gold for Every Emergency*) in 652. He gave special attention to the treatment of women and children with his first three volumes devoted to women's care and the next two about infants and breastfeeding. His Taijiao text includes month-by-month prescriptions for the development of the fetus. He gave instructions on what to eat and what not to eat, and wrote, for example, that eating mule meat during pregnancy may lead to a difficult labor, and that a woman should eat nourishing and easily digestible foods such as meat, fish, and eggs. The text was originally written by Xu Zhicai, a physician who lived before Sun Simiao's time (from around 493–572), but was greatly expanded on by Sun Simiao. Xu Zhicai wrote that if a woman wants a good-looking child, she should feast her eyes on beautiful jade, and for a good-hearted child, she should spend as much time as possible sitting quietly (Maciocia 1998). These are also almost identical to the prescriptions that were found in the *Taichanshu* at the Mawangdui archeological site. Although there is a roughly 700-year difference in the ages of the documents, the information is remarkably identical, without any mention of the *Taichanshu* in Xu Zhicai's or Sun Simiao's prescriptions.

The *Ishimpo* (*Prescriptions from the Heart of Medicine*) is the oldest surviving Japanese medical text, and is 30 volumes in length. It dates to 984 and was written by Tanba no Yasuyori, an acupuncturist at the Japanese court. Although found in Japan, it contains a collection of Chinese medical texts, and is almost identical to the fetal education, month-by-month prescriptions found in Sun Simiao's *Bei Ji Qian Jin Yao Fang* (*Prescriptions Worth a Thousand in Gold for Every Emergency*). It outlines the sequential process, indicating foods that are contraindicated in certain months, plus which channels of the body to avoid needling or applying moxibustion to during acupuncture treatment.

Taijiao had textual parallels between the above-mentioned documents and was literally transmitted from the 2nd to the 10th century. This information was considered so important at the time, and really points to the awareness that the health of the community—and, to a greater context, the country—depended on how well the mother was taken care of throughout her pregnancy, and how her physical and mental health could affect the fetus. Dr Sabine Wilms[1] teaches that this is absolutely fascinating, "at a time when everything was hand copied and texts were at a premium—so there was an oral transmission—this was really, really, treasured knowledge in this culture" (Wilms and Betts, n.d.).

Though many of the ancient Taijiao prescriptions are seemingly absurd when looked at through the lens of our modern understanding, there is now enough research to back up the foundations of Taijiao. Fundamentally, it is about realizing the importance of the health of the mother in relation to the health of her offspring.

Dietary influence

Poring through the research on this subject, I discovered that there is no shortage of data linking short- and long-term health to the fetal environment. What was deemed optimal through keen observation thousands of years ago (before any internal scans were available, and predating nutritional knowledge) is being increasingly confirmed by modern findings. Taijiao has always taken into consideration a women's diet, stressing the need for warming, nourishing foods, and even giving advice on diet for each month of pregnancy. It is positive to see this kind of "lifestyle advice" being integrated more readily into our Western society. In the book, *The First 1000 Days*, Roger Thurow writes,

> If we want to shape the future, to truly improve the world, we have 1000 days to do it, mother by mother, child by child. For what happens in those 1000 days through pregnancy to the second birthday determines to a large extent the course of a child's life—his or her ability to grow, learn, work, succeed—and, by extension, the long-term health, stability, and prosperity of the society in which that child lives. (2016, p.7)

TCM couldn't agree more.

The placenta, in Western medicine, used to be thought of as an impervious barrier. Because of this, drugs were not tested for any harmful effects to the fetus. Thalidomide was one such drug; it caused a watershed event that woke the world up to the fact that the mother's blood and other substances *do* pass through the placenta. Many babies whose mothers took

---

1   Dr Wilms has a PhD in East Asian Studies and Medical Anthropology, and is author of more than a dozen books on Chinese Medicine.

thalidomide to help with sleep and morning sickness were born in the early 1960s with deformities caused by the drug passing through to the developing fetus in utero.

Another unexpected "natural experiment" that predated the thalidomide births occurred in the Netherlands in the 1940s due to the very terrible circumstances of the Second World War. Food supplies became scarce due to a food embargo, resulting in starvation and malnutrition in the Dutch population, known as the "Dutch Hunger Winter." This was a unique chance to study the effects of malnutrition on the fetus in a normally healthy population. Children born just before or just after the embargo could be compared to children born during the famine. Dr Tessa Roseboom, a medical faculty member from the University of Amsterdam, has tracked down the children born during the famine, following them into adulthood. Her research discovered that glucose intolerance occurred with exposure to famine in any of the three trimesters, resulting in health issues later in life (Roseboom et al. 2001). These babies thought they would be born into a world with scarce food, so their bodies became programmed to do well with limited nutrition; instead, they were born into a world in which they could eat whatever they wanted. Because of this, the babies had higher risks of developing cardiovascular disease as adults, problems with gaining weight easily, increased risk of high blood pressure as adults, and many eventually developed type 2 diabetes. Each trimester has its own developmental role for the fetus, so depending on which trimester the mothers experienced malnutrition, health outcomes differed for the babies.

It is interesting to note that researchers have discovered transgenerational effects in babies born from parents who had been in utero during the "Dutch Hunger Winter." The study discovered that women who were in utero during the Dutch famine had higher likelihoods of having babies with neonatal adiposity and poorer health in later life. They posit that:

> In India, currently transitioning to food abundance after generations of poor nutrition, babies are light and small at birth but have increased neonatal adiposity (Stein et al. 2007) compared with European babies. Our findings may indicate that increased neonatal adiposity, and possibly increased diabetes risk, is the direct result of poor maternal nutrition, which occurred generations ago. Public health strategies that focus on improved maternal nutrition during gestation may provide a means of promoting cardiovascular and metabolic health, which will benefit generations to come. (Painter et al. 2008, p.1248)

Grandmaternal stress or malnutrition and its transgenerational epigenetic susceptibility to disease is now being studied extensively as this has obvious long-term medical and public health implications.

The "Dutch Hunger Winter" was tragic, and starvation in our Western world is thankfully not something we need to worry about. Malnutrition, on the other hand, is prevalent today in the form of empty calories from junk food—sugar, salt, and processed foods—contributing to obesity and ill health. Often referred to as the double burden of malnutrition, obesity and undernourishment can co-exist, and the person may still be deficient in micronutrients required for optimal health (*The Lancet* 2019). Just because a diet is high in calories does not mean that the body is not starving in another form. The "Dutch Hunger Winter" research project highlights the importance of obtaining proper nutrition during pregnancy. This has always been one of the cornerstones of Taijiao—a proper diet. But what does this look like in the 21st century?

Sugar

Sugar is high in calories and offers few to zero nutrients. Maternal hyperglycemia, an excess of glucose sugar in the bloodstream during pregnancy, causes metabolic problems (a group of medical problems that put children at risk for heart disease and type 2 diabetes as adults) in children beginning even in early childhood (Boney *et al.* 2005; Hillier *et al.* 2007). Women with high fasting blood sugars were also found to be at a higher risk of high blood pressure during pregnancy and had a higher risk for complications during labor, such as needing an induction, having pre-term labor, or requiring a caesarean section. The adverse outcomes persisted even when they were given drugs such as metformin or insulin to control blood sugar levels (Kaul 2019).

The amount of hidden sugar in foods is staggering. When teaching Taijiao practices, I believe an important modern-day aspect is discussing the recommended upper daily limit of sugar with clients. Labels read differently depending on which part of the world you live in. For example, the serving size of a breakfast food in Canada may be given as ¾ of a cup (29 grams) at 9 grams of sugar per serving. I believe most adults would eat at least one cup (of cereal), bringing the total sugar count to 12 grams. The World Health Organization (WHO) recommends that total free sugars make up less than 5 percent of a woman's daily energy intake. For an average intake of 2000 calories, this would equate to about 25 grams, or 6–7 teaspoons, which is not very much when you consider that many granola bars come in at around 10 grams (just under half the daily limit) of sugar. Hidden sugars in foods such as salad dressings, tomato sauces, sports rehydration drinks, and store-bought coleslaws aren't always considered and can unwittingly contribute many extra teaspoons of sugar per day.

The US[2] and Canada[3] are currently in the process of changing nutrition labels to reflect the daily percentage of sugar added to products; this will make it easier to understand how much added sugar a particular product is contributing to a person's recommended upper daily amount.

Sugar is found in varying amounts in nearly all processed foods: salad dressings, tomato sauces, salsas, yoghurt, granola bars, crackers, etc. The amount of sugar can quickly add up with the abundance of processed foods available to us out there.

High maternal sugar intake may also be associated with the development of allergic asthma and atopy. Queen Mary University of London conducted an observational study between 9000 mother–child pairs to assess the impact of maternal sugar intake on respiratory and allergic outcomes in the children. The mothers, who were in the last trimester of pregnancy, had their total free sugar intake calculated, comprising of sugars added to food or drinks by the manufacturer, cook, or consumer and sugars found naturally in honey, syrups, and unsweetened fruit juice. The verdict was that higher maternal sugar might increase the risk of allergy and allergic asthma in their children. The researchers speculated that the associations could be explained by the high amount of fructose causing a persistent postnatal allergic immune response leading to allergic inflammation in the developing lung. They are urgently following up on this study to investigate their hypothesis further to find out if they can replicate these findings in a different cohort of mothers and children and prevent childhood allergy and allergic asthma. In the meantime, they strongly urge women to reduce free sugar intake in their maternal diet (Bédard *et al.* 2017).

Another study carried out in Korea examined the potential link between perinatal dietary habits and the onset of food allergies. It concluded that a confectionary diet high in baked goods and sugary products may lead to the development of food allergies in children (Kim *et al.* 2019).

The European Academy of Allergy and Clinical Immunology estimate that by 2025, more than 50 percent of all Europeans will suffer from at least

---

2 www.fda.gov/food/nutrition-education-resources-materials/new-nutrition-facts-label
3 www.canada.ca/en/health-canada/services/food-labelling-changes.html

one type of allergy (EAACI 2015). There are many different hypotheses for this, including the increased use of antibiotics, the hygiene hypotheses (we are *too* clean and sanitized), and changes in the diversity of our gut microbiota (as discussed in the next chapter), to name but a few. Avoidance of potentially allergenic foods in the first years of life was originally believed to be a way to avert the development of food allergies. This has not proved helpful, and in countries where dietary avoidance was practiced, food allergies have continued to rise. Some mothers have also tried to eliminate one or more food allergens from their diet during pregnancy in the hope this would reduce the chances of their baby developing an allergy to those foods. Some of these mothers already had a child with food allergies and thought an elimination diet might help. What the research showed, though, is that food elimination during the prenatal period *increased* the odds for the babies to develop an allergy (Robbins *et al.* 2018).

TCM knows that an excess amount of sugar in the diet leads to Spleen *Qi* deficiency and dampness accumulation. A weak Spleen *Qi* will not be able to as effectively transform or transport nutrients to the rest of the body or the fetus, thus leading to a form of malnutrition. Dampness can lead to water metabolism problems, edema, phlegm, and potentially high blood pressure. It can be difficult to reduce excess sugar intake—the more sugar eaten, the more is craved. We can, however, encourage pregnant women to increase naturally sweet foods in their diets, that is, fruit, whole grains, legumes, squash, and carbohydrate-rich vegetables, to satisfy the sweet cravings, nourish their Spleens, and ease the dependence on free sugars.

Influence of stress

There is no denying the effects that stress has on a developing fetus. I include some thoughts on stress here because the mental and physical aspects of Taijiao are considered just as important as the dietary aspects. Plus, there is a tendency to make poor nutritional choices when we're too busy and feeling stressed and overwhelmed. Conveying to pregnant patients the importance and benefit to themselves and their babies of incorporating more "*Yin* time" into their lives—enjoying peaceful surroundings, taking scenic walks in nature, reading uplifting and inspiring content, maintaining peace and calm, and avoiding violent images (the news!) and words—are considered important in Taijiao to help the baby become a well-rounded person. Current research supports the view that reducing stress during pregnancy has a positive impact on the developing fetus. The potential for negative outcomes for the fetus from a mother's high stress load is there, and any lifestyle changes that can be made during the gestational period to reduce this stress load is warranted.

Unfortunately, there is a lot of pressure for pregnant women to continue to live their lives exactly as they were living pre-conception. Days and hours spent working often remain unchanged, and the day-to-day household chores and running errands also remain the same. It is not uncommon to continuing working up to as close to the due date as possible. Most often this is self-determined. There is no definitive answer to how much is too much, and our role as practitioners is to educate our clients while removing any judgment towards someone's opinion and situation. There's a fine line to be walked in certain circumstances—knowing stress should be reduced during pregnancy but then not being able to access the resources or tools that would facilitate this reduction could create a cycle of more stress about being stressed, which we know is counterproductive. I explain further along a mindset shift that helps to transform the effects of stress from adverse to favorable, which is a great place to start.

The term "fetal programming" also applies here—the pernicious role that maternal stress, anxiety, and depression have on the neurodevelopmental outcome for the child is inextricably linked (Hobel, Goldstein, and Barrett 2008). High levels of stress during gestation cause higher rates of pre-term labor and reduced birth weight (Rakers *et al.* 2017). Long term, the effects of stress passed in utero are seen to increase the individual's risk of developing neuropsychiatric, cardiovascular, and metabolic disease in later life (Harris and Seckl 2011). Longitudinal research suggests that pregnant women in the top 15 percent for prenatal anxiety and depression have offspring with about double the increased risk for a mental disorder (for example, attention deficit hyperactivity disorder (ADHD) or anxiety), and this effect extends from childhood through to adolescence (Glover *et al.* 2018).

Dr Nadine Provençal, at the BC Children's Hospital, exposed human neurons to high levels of stress that might be experienced by the fetal brain during times of prenatal stress (Provençal *et al.* 2019). In a 2019 media release she said, "The prenatal period is one of the most dynamic and sensitive periods in a person's life."[4] Her team discovered that developing neurons exposed to stress had epigenetic marks on their genes that endured even after the stress hormones were removed. The mature neurons were also

---

4   www.sfu.ca/university-communications/media-releases/2019/08/stressed-out--new-research-on-prenatal-stress-exposure-could-exp.html#:~:text=%E2%80%9CThe%20prenatal%20period%20is%20one,also%20impact%20her%20developing%20fetus

much more sensitive to future stress due to these original epigenetic marks created from the stress. The researchers then took these findings out of the lab to study the umbilical cords of newborns exposed to maternal stress, including maternal depression and anxiety. They found the same epigenetic marks in a newborn's genes that had been exposed to maternal stress, proving the results in the lab translated to real life (Provençal *et al.* 2019). It is still not 100 percent understood how or why stress might have these long-term impacts on a developing fetus, and research is still underway.

There are two kinds of stress, objective and subjective. Subjective stress is not easily measured—it is a personal reaction to the stressor. We all respond differently to stress and when we *perceive* stress to be negative, it is this perception that causes the negative effects in the body (Keller *et al.* 2012). The more someone *believes* the stress in their lives is harmful, the more it is! Objective stress, on the other hand, uses measurements and refers to the amount of hardship someone is subjected to during a stressful time—the amount of days, how much it affects their life, and the losses they may incur due to the stress, that is, money, property, family. These are quantifiable, and for the purpose of maternal research can clearly show the effects of stress on the fetus and why pregnant women should be well taken care of, especially during an emergency.

Project Ice Storm was able to take an extremely stressful event, with quantifiable measures, and measure objective stress in relation to fetal outcomes. It was started in 1998 during an ice storm in Québec, Canada, which left millions without electricity for up to 40 days during the coldest part of the year. There were, of course, many pregnant women who experienced this stressful event. Researchers had a great opportunity to study the repercussions on the children as they have grown up. They continue to this day to study the effects that this natural disaster has had on the fetuses in utero. The babies born after the ice storm are now in their early 20s, and the research shows negative changes in cognitive (King and Laplante 2005), linguistic (Laplante *et al.* 2008), immunological (Turcotte-Tremblay *et al.* 2014), motor (Cao *et al.* 2014), and behavioral outcomes (Veru *et al.* 2015) in the growing children. Just over 20 years since the ice storm, the research has shown that the children whose mothers had a higher amount of prenatal objective stress (for example, days without power) had lower IQs than the children whose mothers experienced less objective stress. The more difficult the hardship, the higher the girls' body mass index at age 5.5, and the more predictive it was of an earlier puberty (Duchesne *et al.* 2017). "If there's anything that we all agree on, it's that the fetus is incredibly vulnerable and fragile, and that even subtle perturbations in the mother's mood or her objective circumstances can have measurable effects on the fetus that last for years," explained Suzanne King, a professor of psychiatry at McGill University and lead investigator for Project Ice Storm (quoted in Bielski 2009).

Antenatal stress can also influence childhood asthma and atopic diseases, linked by a shared underlying problem with the immune system, such as eczema, allergic rhinitis, and asthma or food allergies (Andersson et al. 2016; van de Loo et al. 2016). The studies that were included in these systemic reviews suggested a relationship between maternal stress and atopic and allergic disorders in children. They all had the mothers self-report their degrees of stress (subjective stress) in relationship to negative life events, anxiety/depression, bereavement, and distress and job strain. What these studies didn't include were the women's dietary habits. My hunch is that when levels of perceived stress were higher, this would also have shifted food choices, potentially increasing sugar intake, which would link with the previously mentioned studies on excess maternal sugar and atopy.

It has been documented that chronic stress exposure affects the brain's response to food. When stressed, it is easier to reach for sweet, salty "comfort" snacks (cookies, chips, chocolate cake, candy bars, crackers, etc.) and can be a predisposition for obesogenic eating (Tryon et al. 2013). We know from the research mentioned previously in regards to stress perception that as long as the stress isn't related to poverty, abuse, or neglect (which would require community or government support outside of our practice), research shows that if there is a belief and a mindset that stress isn't harmful, then our bodies respond and can thrive under stress, producing a beneficial cascade of hormones. A negative mindset towards stress can instead cause burnout and depression. In addition to using stress reduction strategies (yoga, deep breathing, mindfulness practice, walking in nature, acupuncture, massage, music, etc.), employing a growth mindset towards stress—believing that stress in our lives is a challenge that lifts us to a higher level of energy and performance to help us cope—is another tool to help our pregnant clients nurture their fetuses.

A body under stress has just as much of an impact on the developing fetus as maternal diet and nutrition. This is my motivation for having included it here alongside children's dietary therapy. Let us all share and teach mindfulness in terms of diet, lifestyle, sleep quality, and work–life balance during pregnancy, with the intention of increasing health outcomes for the newborn. It is hard for feelings of overwhelm, anxiety, and depression to co-exist when there is a harmonious body/mind/spirit.

Bringing Taijiao into our modern-day lives

The recommendations below are all intended to help support and nourish a fetus's growth through to labor. The time in the womb is the first opportunity to begin nurturing a child's growth and health.

Recommendations for the first trimester

There are a lot of changes happening in the body in the first trimester and it is common for women to feel fatigued and easily nauseous or to vomit. TCM encourages rest, napping, and a warming, cooked and nourishing diet.

- **Minimize salads, raw vegetables, and chilled, iced, or frozen foods** to support Spleen *Qi*, Blood nourishment, and digestion.
- **Eat as much as possible in season and grown locally** to stay in seasonal attunement and to get the most nutrients out of the food. Fruit and vegetables that have travelled long distances and that have been stored can lose a lot of their vitamin content (Rickman, Bruhn, and Barrett 2007).
- **Eat plenty of folate-rich foods**, such as leafy green vegetables, lentils, black beans, asparagus, peas, and broccoli. All women are recommended to take a folic acid supplement (600 micrograms per day) before and during pregnancy to prevent birth defects.
- **Keep free sugars to a minimum** and instead incorporate fruits, carbohydrate-rich vegetables, and whole grains.
- **For morning sickness, eat smaller, more frequent meals**, with a little bit of protein at each meal. Staying hydrated is also important, as dehydration will worsen the nausea. Sipping small amounts of water may be easier than a full cup at a time. Ginger has been traditionally used for nausea—up to three cups per day, as it is heating (see the recipe for Ginger (or Scallion (spring onion)) Tea).
- **Light exercise**, if any, is indicated at this stage. Keep the body at an even temperature with no extremes of hot or cold. Watch out for saunas and hot tubs, hot yoga, strenuous exercise, hot baths (warm is okay), electric blankets on the stomach or low back area, and cold drafts on the lower back or abdomen.

- **Barley** has traditionally been recommended in TCM for pregnancy, and is especially beneficial in the first trimester. It is cooling, nourishes *Yin*, tonifies *Qi* and Blood, harmonizes the Stomach, and is easy to digest. Drinking Barley Water has the additional bonus of easing nausea (see below).

Barley Water
Ingredients

- ¾ cup of pearl barley
- 6 cups of water
- Optional: Honey to taste (enters all the *Yin* organs)

Method

1. Rinse the pearl barley in a sieve under cold water until the water runs clear.
2. Place the pearl barley in a saucepan with water. Bring to a boil, then reduce the heat to a simmer.
3. Simmer for 30 minutes.
4. Drink plain or sweeten with honey to your liking. Eat the cooked pearl barley as a porridge.

BENEFICIAL FOODS TO INCORPORATE DURING PREGNANCY

Below is a list of some beneficial foods to incorporate during pregnancy. This list is not exhaustive, and a varied and diverse diet including local, seasonal produce is highly recommended. These foods are great at building Blood and *Yin* to prevent anemia and for nourishing *Qi*, which will aid digestion and help with overall energy and the rapid growth and development of the baby.

- **Amaranth:** cooling thermal nature; sweet and bitter flavor. Tonifies *Qi*; clears Liver fire; drains dampness; regulates water metabolism. Highly nourishing for pregnant women.
- **Apples:** cooling thermal nature; sweet and bitter flavor. Nourish the Lungs; tonify *Qi*, Liver, and Intestines; soothe indigestion.
- **Asparagus:** cooling thermal nature; sweet and bitter flavor. Tonifies Kidney *Yin*; resolves dampness; helps with water metabolism. High

in vitamin K, which helps to transport calcium throughout the body. Aids fetal bone development and folate, which helps to prevent neural tube defects.

- **Black beans:** neutral thermal nature; sweet flavor. Tonify Spleen and Kidneys; nourish the Blood and *Yin*. High in folate, which helps to prevent neural tube defects.

- **Bone broths (chicken and beef):** warming thermal nature; sweet flavor. Nourish Essence; tonify Defensive *Qi* (*Wei Qi*); benefit digestion.

- **Broccoli:** cooling thermal nature; sweet, pungent, slightly bitter flavor. Clears heat; regulates water metabolism.

- **Carrots:** neutral thermal nature; sweet flavor. Tonify Spleen and Stomach; tonify *Qi*; clear heat; resolve dampness. Increase milk production for nursing.

- **Cherries:** warming thermal nature; sweet flavor. Tonify the Spleen; rich in iron so great for anemia and tonifying the Blood.

- **Chickpeas (garbanzo beans):** neutral thermal nature; sweet flavor. Tonify Spleen *Qi*, Stomach, and Heart.

- **Collard greens:** neutral to warming thermal nature. Nourish Liver *Yin* and Blood. Highest plant source of calcium.

- **Grapes:** neutral thermal nature; sweet and sour flavor. Enter all the *Yin* organs; tonify *Qi* and the Blood; purify the Blood; help with water metabolism.

- **Green peas:** neutral thermal nature; sweet flavor. Tonify Spleen and Stomach; harmonize digestion; calm an overworked Liver. Help to move the *Qi* in the right direction for digestion, which is downwards. Good for GERD (gastroesophageal reflux disease), vomit, and belching.

- **Hormone and antibiotic-free beef (free range and organic is preferable):** neutral to warming thermal nature; sweet flavor. Tonifies *Qi* and the Blood. Moderate amounts as too much creates dampness in the body.

- **Hormone and antibiotic-free chicken (free range and organic is preferable):** warming thermal nature; sweet flavor. Tonifies *Qi* and the Blood; nourishes the Essence and marrow; warms the body. Moderate amounts as too much creates dampness in the body.

- **Kiwifruit:** cooling thermal nature, sweet and sour flavor. Clear heat. Beneficial for constipation.

- **Lentils:** neutral thermal nature; sweet flavor. Regulate water metabolism; tonify Kidney Essence. High in iron and folate, which helps to prevent neural tube defects.

- **Millet:** cooling thermal nature; sweet and salty flavor. Tonifies Kidney *Yin*; harmonizes the Spleen and Stomach; nourishes *Yin*; clears heat. Prevents miscarriage and eases morning sickness.
- **Oats:** warming thermal nature; sweet and slightly bitter flavor. Tonify Spleen *Qi* and the Blood.
- **Organic eggs:** neutral thermal nature; sweet flavor. Tonify Blood and *Yin*; nourish Essence. Contain choline, an important nutrient responsible for brain development in babies.
- **Potatoes:** neutral thermal nature; sweet flavor. Tonify *Qi*; moisten the Intestines; nourish the Spleen and Stomach. A plain boiled potato is quite easy to digest.
- **Pumpkin:** cooling thermal nature; sweet and slightly bitter flavor. Great for pregnancy as it helps to regulate blood sugar, calms the fetus, and promotes lactation. Removes excess damp and helps to clear mucus and phlegm from the Lungs.
- **Quinoa:** warming thermal nature; sweet and sour flavor. Nourishes the whole body, especially Kidney *Yang* and the Pericardium. A complete protein.
- **Sardines:** neutral thermal nature; sweet and salty flavor. Tonify *Qi*, *Yin*, and the Blood. Regulate water metabolism in the body. High in Omega-3 fatty acids, which benefit pregnancy and the developing fetus.
- **Shiitake mushrooms:** neutral thermal nature; sweet flavor. Tonify *Qi*, the Blood, and Defensive *Qi*; resolve phlegm. Antibacterial and antiviral effects in the body. Great for helping immunity.
- **Soybeans (non-GMO):** neutral to cooling thermal nature; sweet flavor. Clear heat; tonify the Spleen and Kidneys, *Qi*, Blood, and *Yin*. Helps to remove excess fluid during pregnancy and is helpful for toxemia. Increase milk production for nursing.
- **Spinach:** cooling thermal nature; sweet and bitter flavor. Nourishes and clears heat from the Blood. Has a moistening effect on the Intestines and is therefore great for constipation. Not recommended for anyone with loose stools.
- **Strawberries:** cooling thermal nature; sweet and sour flavor. Tonify *Yin* and the Blood; enter all the *Yin* organs. Improve appetite.
- **Sweet potatoes:** neutral thermal nature; sweet flavor. Tonify the

Spleen and Stomach; build *Qi*, Blood, and *Yin*. Also abundant in vitamin B6.

- **Vegetable broths:** warming thermal nature. Tonify Defensive *Qi*; benefit digestion.
- **Wild salmon:** warming thermal nature; sweet flavor. Tonifies the Spleen and Stomach; nourishes *Qi* and the Blood. High in vitamin B6 to help with morning sickness. High in Omega-3 fatty acids, which benefit pregnancy and the developing fetus.
- **Winter squash:** warming thermal nature; sweet flavor. Tonifies the Spleen and Stomach; tonifies *Qi*; removes excess damp. Terrific at strengthening the digestive system.
- **Yams:** neutral thermal nature; sweet flavor. Tonify the Spleen, Stomach, Lung *Qi*, and *Yin*; nourish the *Yin* of the Kidneys and retain *Jing*. Contain an abundant amount of vitamin B6, which is helpful for morning sickness.

Seafood consumption is connected to beneficial associations in neurocognitive development in infants and adolescents. In other words, it has been found to be beneficial in improving memory, thinking, reasoning, attention, judgment, mental imagery, language, solving problems, and creativity, to name just some of the cognitive functions. A systemic review found that children of mothers not eating oily seafood had about three times a greater risk of hyperactivity (Hibbeln *et al.* 2019). The benefits of seafood are obtained if over 4 ounces and up to 12 ounces per week are eaten, due to the Omega-3 fatty acids, which are divided into DHA (docosahexaenoic) and EPA (eicosapentaenoic). Some of the women in the study were eating upwards of 100 ounces of fish per week. Although there were no adverse effects to fetal neurocognitive development recorded due to the higher mercury consumption, it is still advisable to remain within the government-recommended amounts, which differ from country to country. The Environmental Working Group (EWG) has calculated the levels of mercury found in different types of seafood, and offers consumption guidelines[5] on its website based on different factors such as weight and whether someone is pregnant or not. It lists fish that have the lowest mercury counts, are sustainable, and suggests the ocean from which the fish are most optimally harvested.

Pregnant women on a vegetarian diet can eat **plant-based sources of Omega-3** instead. Seaweed and algae both contain *preformed* DHA and

---

5   ee www.ewg.org/consumer-guides

EPA, which means that the body doesn't need to convert it into these substances. These are good sources. The other plant-based sources, such as flax seeds, chia seeds, walnuts, hemp seeds, kale, and spinach, although extremely healthy, do not contain preformed DHA and EPA. Instead, they contain ALA (alpha-lipoic acid), which the body must then *convert* into EPA and DHA. This conversion process is inefficient and only a small percentage of the ALA gets converted while the rest is either stored or used as immediate energy, like other fats. The actual Omega-3 absorbed by the body is quite low. To be certain that the developing fetus can obtain the Omega-3 required for optimal neurodevelopment, taking a supplement in the form of algal oil (also known as algae oil) derived from algae and a plant-based source of EPA and DHA is highly recommended.

Minimize the amount of heating, drying, and pungent foods. A woman's body "heats up" during the first trimester due to the increase in Blood volume. Blood volume starts to increase during this time and keeps on expanding until the third trimester. This is an important time to nourish *Yin*—heating and drying foods can burn up *Yin* Fluids and *Yin* Blood if consumed in excess. Pregnancies that have failure of maternal plasma volume expansion (deficient Blood) have been linked to adverse pregnancy outcomes: pre-eclampsia, fetal growth restriction, and pre-term birth.

Examples of heating and pungent foods include:

- Cayenne
- Chili pepper
- Cinnamon bark
- Deep-fried food
- Galangal
- Garlic
- Horseradish
- Lamb
- Shallots
- Smoked foods[6] (salmon, beef)
- Spirits
- Wasabi.

Recommendations for the second and third trimesters

Appetite may be better in these trimesters, with possibly less food aversions. There is more energy in the second trimester, with some fatigue returning in the third due to the extra weight and growth of the baby.

Nourishing the spirit and the mind, taking in a beautiful sunset, reading uplifting and inspirational novels or poetry, absorbing awe-inspiring art, listening to soothing music—these are all beneficial to the fetus in ways we cannot yet fully explain.

Sleep and rest also encourage the formation of Blood and *Yin*. Napping

---

6   Smoking food changes its property to become very heating, as does barbequing the food.

helps to rejuvenate Liver Blood and gives the Kidneys a rest. Pregnancy requires a lot of energy from the Kidneys, as they govern reproduction, and the Kidneys do well with lots of laying down and time spent doing less.

Incorporate relaxation techniques to reduce stress such as meditation, deep breathing, warm baths, walking, spending time in nature, prenatal yoga, prenatal massage, acupuncture, employing positive self-talk, using mantras, and talking to others, whether it be through group pregnancy classes, one-on-one counseling, or with family and friends.

Reframing views on stress will help to alter the effects stress has on the body. Research has shown that how we *view* stress impacts health much more than stress itself (Keller *et al.* 2012). Viewing stress as a helpful rather than harmful part of life is associated with better health and emotional wellbeing, even during periods of high stress. Instead of thinking of stress as the enemy, think of it as something that gets the body energized and ready for action. Stanford researcher, Kelly McGonigal, writes about this in her book, *The Upside of Stress*. She advises,

> They were also taught a three-step process for practicing the new mindset whenever they felt stressed. The first step is to acknowledge stress when you experience it. Simply allow yourself to notice the stress, including how it affects your body. The second step is to welcome the stress by recognizing that it's a response to something you care about. Can you connect to the positive motivation behind the stress? What is at stake here, and why does it matter to you? The third step is to make use of the energy that stress gives you, instead of wasting that energy trying to manage your stress. What can you do right now that reflects your goals and values? (2016, p.29)

The amniotic fluid the baby is marinating in is influenced by what the pregnant mother is eating. Flavors in the mother's diet transfer into the amniotic fluid, which the baby swallows, and by the second trimester the baby begins to taste and recognize foods. Pregnant women who drank 300 milliliters of carrot juice for four days per week for three consecutive weeks in the last trimester and for two months during lactation had babies who preferred carrot-flavored cereal compared with the control group who only drank water—their babies made negative facial expressions when given the same carrot-flavored cereal (Mennella, Jagnow, and Beauchamp 2001). This kind of flavor detection has an evolutionary basis. Flavors that come from the womb represent foods that are safe and available in the environment, and these would be tasted again in breast milk. So, when babies get their "first" bites of food, they will know which flavors have passed the pre-screening, and those foods will get the green light!

Looking at Taijiao through the Five Elements lens

- Wood = Movement.
- Fire = Reframe stress.
- Earth = Nourish with food and connect to the baby.
- Metal = Take in beautiful surroundings, music, and art.
- Water = Rest and meditate.

Zuo Yuezi, "sitting the month"

The first 40-day period after a child is born is considered the Golden Month in TCM and Chinese culture. It's about "mothering the mother" and offering her support and care with nourishing foods and allowing her time to rest and bond with her newborn baby. It is a time for a woman to rest and recuperate following labor; labor is a taxing event that depletes the *Qi* and Blood, while the body is required to produce milk and sustenance for the growing baby, which can leave the body vulnerable to disease. *Yang Qi* is depleted after labor, and so the body is easily cold and needs to be protected: staying home, staying warm, eating warming and bland food, keeping bundled up from drafts, and doing as little physical labor as possible are all meant to strengthen and build *Qi*, Blood, and *Yang*. A study carried out among postpartum women in Taiwan who were "sitting the month" found that they had lower severity of physical symptoms and lower odds of prenatal depression (Chien *et al.* 2006). Breastfeeding is not always an easy endeavor and can feel like a full-time job in the initial weeks. The more support offered to a woman postnatally, be it from her partner, family, or friends, the more she can focus on her health and the health of her baby and breastfeeding. The initial month is a crucial period for establishing milk production and getting the latch down pat. The more energy and time that can go towards focusing on this, the better the chances that breastfeeding will work out. Breastfeeding, when possible, is a child's first best source of dietary therapy.

CHAPTER 4

Populating the Microbiome

All disease begins in the gut.

Hippocrates, 460–375 BCE

In *The Yellow Emperor's Classic of Medicine*, Huang Di teaches,

> In the old days the sages treated disease by preventing illness before it began, just as a good government or emperor was able to take the necessary steps to avert war. Treating an illness after it has begun is like suppressing revolt after it has broken out. If someone digs a well when thirsty, or forges weapons after becoming engaged in battle, one cannot help but ask: Are not these actions too late?

The human microbiome is a vast and dynamic area of research, and there is continually more being discovered and disputed about the 100 trillion different bacteria, microorganisms, viruses, protozoa, and fungi present in the gastrointestinal (GI) tract. The connection of the microbiome to wellbeing and, on the flip side, to disease and malaise, is intriguing and as more is understood, it is found that many diseases (for example, type 2 diabetes, asthma, eczema, and obesity in later life) have their origin in the lack of diverse or not as friendly microbes (Wang *et al.* 2017). Diversity in the microbiome, also known as gut microbial species richness, is used as an indicator to define microbial health. The more bacteria, the merrier! The range of diversity and abundance varies from person to person and it is unknown if there is one specific type of microbiome that is superior to another. This is the reason why the exploding use of antibacterial soaps and cleaners and antibiotics used in the animal food chain is of concern—if diversity equals health, we don't want to be killing off the good with the bad, especially during children's formative years.

The microorganisms in the microbiome have been found to be responsible for providing nutrients and vitamins that our bodies are not normally able to make on their own; they help to digest food and are constantly preventing unwanted foreigners like salmonella or listeria from gaining a foothold.

Science is realizing that the gut microbiota may also play an important role in food allergies. Allergies to foods have been on the rise in children for reasons not yet fully understood, and have a significant impact on the quality of life for children and for their families. Severe food allergic reactions were rare 40 years ago but are now the leading cause of anaphylaxis treated in American Emergency Departments (Sampson 2016).

Scientists at the University of Chicago compared the gut microbiome from healthy babies against the gut microbiome of babies who had an allergy to milk (Feehley *et al.* 2019). They found that their microbiomes differed and the babies with the milk allergy had biomes with unusually adult characteristics. The healthy babies, on the other hand, had higher amounts of one species of bacteria called *Clostridia*, which is a gram-positive, anaerobic, spore-forming class of Firmicutes commonly found in soils and in the microbiota of humans and animals. The bacteria have been found to have protective properties against allergies. *Clostridia* have also been found to have a protective factor against peanut allergy (Stefka *et al.* 2014). The researchers then took samples from both the healthy babies and the babies with a milk allergy and cultivated the digestive tracts of mice that were germ-free (mice bred in isolators to ensure they are blocked from any exposure to microorganisms to keep them free of detectable levels of bacteria and viruses). As they thought, the mice with bacteria from the healthy babies were protected against the milk allergy, whereas the mice colonized with the bacteria from the milk allergy babies developed allergies themselves and contained lower amounts of the protective bacteria *Clostridia* (Feehley *et al.* 2019).

A mother's chronic prenatal psychological stress and elevated hair cortisol levels have been linked with the infant's gut microbiota composition (Aatsinki *et al.* 2020). This may tie in with why chronic stress during pregnancy has been shown to have potential health effects for the infant, such as wheezing and asthma (van de Loo *et al.* 2016), suboptimal emotional, behavioral, and cognitive development (Monk, Lugo-Candelas, and Trumpff 2019; Weinstock 2008), increased odds of personality disorder (Brannigan *et al.* 2020) and impaired development in key brain regions (Lautarescu *et al.* 2019; Wu *et al.* 2020). Higher levels of prenatal stress translated to increased abundances of *Proteobacteria genera* in infant microbiota and lower levels of *Akkermansia genera*, which is considered to promote health, at least for certain adults. *Proteobacteria* contain species that can cause inflammation in the body and may also be associated with a child's disease risk later in life. Low cortisol concentrations (a lower stress indicator) in the mother's hair was linked to increased abundances of *Lactobacillus* in the infant gut microbiota, and these are considered to promote health. The research is in its infancy, but TCM has always linked digestive health to overall mental health and wellbeing. The connection of Spleen *Qi* sending Food *Qi* up to the Heart to make Blood cannot be ignored. Sufficient Blood is needed for a clear mind and an anchor for the *Shen* (spirit), whereas a Blood deficiency can lead to anxiety, insomnia, poor memory, and, in severe cases, mental disorders and psychiatric disease.

Spleen and Stomach *Qi* deficiency mirror symptoms of gut microbial dysbiosis. Defined in its simplest form, gut microbial dysbiosis is the disruption of the complex gut microbial community. Symptoms of gut microbial dysbiosis are digestive disturbances: bloating, diarrhea, constipation, and food sensitivities. These symptoms all point to Spleen and Stomach *Qi* deficiency, and as we know, can be aided through the process of nourishing these organs in TCM. If children are to have healthy Spleen and Stomach *Qi*, then their diet, their time in the womb, and nurturing are all important, of course, but we cannot ignore our 21st-century understanding of the microbiota and the knowledge that the first few years of life may be crucial to the development and populating of our gut microbiomes.

Probiotic supplementation

Taking probiotics has been touted as one of the ways to colonize and improve the microbiome, but most research to date has been inconclusive and contradictory. Marketing of probiotics has outpaced the research. One study by the Weizmann Institute of Science in Israel found that it was better to allow the gut flora to repopulate on its own after a dose of antibiotics rather than taking probiotics, which has become a mainstream antidote (Zmora *et al.* 2018). Surprisingly, the probiotics delayed the normal flora from returning to its pre-antibiotic state for months following treatment, longer than the placebo group, which allowed for spontaneous recovery. They found the best method for returning to a pre-antibiotic state was after an autologous fecal microbiota transplantation (aFMT), which uses the person's individual flora in the transfer; this method was able to restore fecal bacterial richness within eight days. The study differed from others in that it not only looked at stool samples, but it also measured the colonization, or lack thereof, with an upper and lower endoscopy.

Likening to the TCM model, which views everybody as an individual and tailors treatment according to individual signs and symptoms, there is not a one-size-fits-all model when it comes to homeostasis within our gut flora. How can taking a specific probiotic be the answer to digestive issues or to aid in populating a child's gut when we are all so different and are still uncovering this vast community? Could giving children probiotics backfire? These are questions that have yet to be answered, and it may be prudent to avoid the prescribing and use of probiotics until we can be certain of the benefit and even more certain of not causing harm or disruption in the gut. For now, they are deemed "safe" for children, unless the child is immunocompromised.

One recent study showed the potential for harm caused by a probiotic. The study, undertaken by Washington University School of Medicine on mice models, used a common probiotic marketed as an antidiarrheal in Europe. Tests in mice demonstrated how these bacteria evolved in the animals' intestines in a few weeks. In some cases, the strain developed the ability to damage the protective layer of the intestinal tract, which is seen in IBS (Crook *et al.* 2019). What they realized is that these probiotics are living microorganisms that can behave differently depending on someone's current flora, diet, and immune system function.

Some specific strains of probiotics *have* proven to offer positive effects. A systemic review and meta-analysis found a moderate benefit with the strains *Lactobacillus rhamnosus* GG (LGG) and *Saccharomyces boulardii* in aiding the prevention of antibiotic-associated diarrhea (AAD) in children (Blaabjerg, Artzi, and Aabenhus 2017). What the researchers also discovered, though, was that only 18 percent of the studies looked at had a low risk of bias, and those studies did not find a significant reduction in the prevention of AAD. They urged caution in the interpretation of the results, but then also said that their results were in line with a previous Cochrane review (Goldenberg *et al.* 2015) on the prevention of pediatric AAD. It is all enough to make your head spin and your tummy feel queasy!

Many of the studies currently looking at the use of probiotic supplementation are conflicting; until the microbiome is better understood and supplements can be trusted to deliver what they promise on the package, I recommend being wary of giving them to children unless there has been a prescription for a specific reason. The microbiome has come this far in human history without the need for probiotic pills.

Diet and the microbiome

Nature knows best, and food-based probiotics contain microorganisms that have greater bacterial diversity than over-the-counter probiotics and in amounts highly exceeding supplements for a fraction of the cost. Fermentation and pickling have been used to preserve food for thousands of years and are a component in every traditional culture's diets. Some examples include Amazake, a fermented rice beverage from Japan, Garri, a popular West African food made from cassava tubers, and Atchara, a traditional pickling of green papaya. Food is eaten fresh when it is in season and the rest is fermented so it can be eaten during the rest of the year. Not all fermented foods are a source of probiotics (beer and wine are ferments but do not contain live probiotics after the fermentation process), but some of the more commonly found probiotic-containing foods are:

- Cheese (raw, unpasteurized—Gruyère, Emmental, Edam, Cheddar, Feta, and Gouda are some common probiotic varieties).
- European-style dry fermented sausage.
- Kefir (use unsweetened).
- Nonheated sauerkraut and kimchee (unpasteurized).
- Pickled vegetables (need to be traditionally pickled without the use of vinegar or heat to offer probiotics).
- Yoghurt.

Also, simply eating produce may be key to obtaining probiotics in our diet, not through expensive supplementation. And, according to the apple research reported below, freshly harvested, organically managed produce may be the most optimal. An apple contains about 100 million bacteria, which are found mostly inside, in the core (which I will admit I have never eaten but will now consider doing) containing 90 percent of the bacteria (Wassermann, Müller, and Berg 2019). The seeds have the most microbes, and although they contain trace amounts of cyanide, one core per day is fine for adults. Children would probably not enjoy the seed anyway, and these could be removed for them from the core. The freshly harvested, organically managed apples harbor a significantly more diverse and distinct microbiota compared to conventional ones, by a 40 percent difference. "*Escherichia Shigella*, a group of bacteria that includes known pathogens, was found in most of the conventional apple samples, but none from the organic apples. For beneficial *Lactobacilli*—of probiotic fame—the reverse was true," says study senior author Professor Gabriele Berg, of Graz University of Technology, Austria (Wassermann *et al.* 2019). The organic apples had more health-promoting bacteria, whereas the opposite was true of the conventionally grown varieties.

Prebiotics are functional, typically nondigestible food components that help the growth and activity of specific groups of bacteria in the gut. They feed the intestinal microbiota and their digestive byproducts are short-chain fatty acids (SCFAs), which include acetate, propionate, and butyrate, that are released into the Blood circulation and affect not only the GI tract but also distant organs. SCFAs have been implicated in health benefits such as reduced inflammatory disease, cardiovascular disease, and diabetes (De Filippis *et al.* 2015). All prebiotics are a form of fiber, but not all fiber is considered a prebiotic. Breast milk contains oligosaccharides, which are an early source of prebiotics; many infant formulas are now adding some oligosaccharides found in breast milk to bring infant formula closer in composition to human milk.

Fiber found in fruit, vegetables and legumes, whole grains, and nuts has been associated with greater microbial diversity and is therefore important to include in children's diets (Simpson and Campbell 2015). Increased dietary diversity has also been linked to a reduction in food allergies, possibly because of the exposure the GI microbiota gets to a diverse range of foods and nutrients (Venter *et al.* 2020).

The foods listed below contain prebiotics:

- **Fruit:** apples, grapefruit, kiwifruit, nectarines, persimmons, pomegranate, watermelon, white peaches; also dried fruit (e.g., dates, figs).
- **Grains:** barley, oats, rye, wheat.
- **Legumes:** baked beans, chickpeas, lentils, red kidney beans, soybeans.
- **Nuts:** almonds, cashews, pistachios.
- **Vegetables:** artichokes, asparagus, beetroot, chicory, dandelion greens, fennel bulbs, garlic, green peas, leeks, onions, savoy cabbage, shallots, snow peas, spring onions, sweetcorn.
- **Other:** cocoa, flax seeds, seaweed, honey, acacia gum.

Caesarean sections

Researchers in the Baby Biome Study, a large-scale UK birth cohort study and biobank, published the largest ever study of neonatal microbiomes in 2019. Their discovery? Babies born naturally acquire bacteria found in their mother's gut bacteria whereas babies born by caesarean section (C-section) are colonized by "opportunistic pathogens" residing in hospital settings

(Shao *et al.* 2019). These "opportunistic pathogens" may be one of the reasons posited that babies born by C-section have alarmingly higher rates of asthma, eczema, and other allergic conditions than babies born vaginally.

There is such a marked difference between the microbiome when born by C-section that researchers in the Baby Biome Study said they would be able to tell you how a baby had been born just by looking at their fecal sample! By around nine months of age the microbiomes of C-section babies did start to resemble vaginally born babies, but those first nine months are a crucial formation period for the immune system, and researchers believe that the right microbes might not be there to train the immune system properly. "The studies in our lab—and the labs of several other researchers—prove that microbes really do impact a child's health. What shocked us most was how early this starts—the first one hundred days of life are critical. We knew microbes played a role in well-being, but we had no idea how soon this role began," write Dr B. Brett Finlay and Dr Marie-Claire Arrieta, authors of *Let Them Eat Dirt: Saving Your Child from an Oversanitized World (2016, p xii).*

C-sections are life-saving, for both the mother and the baby, and as any woman who has given birth knows, when it comes to laboring, things may not and often do not go as planned. C-sections are critical in these emergency situations when there is a prolonged labor, fetal distress, placenta problems, carrying multiples or abnormal positioning, and for women with chronic health conditions such as heart disease, high blood pressure, or gestational diabetes. If the pregnancy is healthy and there are no medical reasons for a C-section, vaginal births offer the best outcome for babies, especially regarding their microbiome. After a C-section, babies are often whisked away for testing to make sure they are healthy and well post-surgery, and they do not get the initial skin-to-skin care (SSC). SSC involves placing an unclothed newborn chest-to-chest with their mother for one hour post-birth, and is one of the most effective methods for promoting exclusive breastfeeding. Breastfeeding offers benefits to the microbial seeding process in infants and is also the best food for babies in the first year of life. Many hospitals are now allowing and offering the set-up for SSC after a C-section birth, and this can be discussed with doctors prior to a planned C-section birth. This is one way of aiding the microbiome for babies born by C-section; another way, as discussed below, seems to be by taking a walk in a park...with a furry friend!

Breast milk

TCM has ways of helping women who may have low milk supply, or engorgement or mastitis, through herbs, acupuncture, and lifestyle advice. As we understand more about the role breastfeeding plays in the seeding of the infant microbiome, it is really important for women to get off to a good breastfeeding start. The benefits of breastfeeding are multitudinous, and most women have the desire to breastfeed their infant. It can be a difficult endeavor, though, especially for first-time mothers; latching, milk supply, sore nipples, and the round-the-clock feeding schedule can seem insurmountable. Fortunately there is a lot of support available to women, through La Leche Leagues, community nurses, lactation consultants, hospital-grade breast pumps, and our own medicine (TCM), when we are knowledgeable in the diagnosis and treatment methods.

Breast milk is teeming with live bacteria that colonize the infant's gut. Certain bacteria co-occur in the mother's milk and their infant's stool with exclusive breastfeeding (Differding *et al.* 2020). Breast milk is made from the mother's Blood, which is another reason why in TCM the "Golden Month" postnatally is a way for the mother to rebuild her *Qi* and Blood and ensure that milk supply is established.

Green space and a pet in the home

When breastfeeding is not an option, following a C-section birth, or when given antibiotics during birth, researchers have discovered other ways that help populate the microbiome in infants. Nature-related intervention, along with having a pet in the home, are both showing promising results. Having a furry friend living in the home during the second and third trimester of pregnancy as well as three months after birth increased the abundance of *Ruminococcus* and *Oscillospira* bacteria by double in the babies' guts; these are two microbes that have been shown to be associated with reduced childhood metabolic and allergic disease (Tun *et al.* 2017). The pets in the study consisted of dogs, cats, or a cat *and* a dog. Pet exposure was also linked to lower levels of enterobacteria—associated with salmonella or other infections—in C-section babies who normally have high levels of these microbes by three months of age. This study was not a controlled experiment and cannot say for certain that pets equal better health for children, but it does show that pets help the diversity and richness of the gut flora.

A team of Swedish scientists used national registries for one million

Swedish children, and they found that children who grew up with a dog had a 15 percent less chance of developing asthma (Fall *et al.* 2015).

Trees, soil, grass, and plants might offer another remedy. Infants who were formula-fed but lived within 500 meters of a natural environment had a microbiome that was similar to a breast-fed baby, and if there was a pet in the home, it was an even closer match. Although not exactly sure of the mechanisms, the researchers believe this is because if you live in a high-rise flat but own a dog, you will regularly use the natural spaces near your home, and the dog acts like a conduit (Nielsen *et al.* 2020). Researcher Anita Kozyrskyj, Pediatrics Professor at the University of Alberta, says she often receives emails from new mothers who are unable to breastfeed and who are concerned about their child's futures (see Rutherford 2020). Based on the results of her study she will advise them to take their babies out to natural environments and to consider getting a pet. Who knows, this may even lead to clinics offering doggy snuggle time for babies to help them acquire the disease-protecting bacteria offered by animals!

Antibiotics

Antibiotics are unfortunately one of the most prescribed medications for children, including infants, in the Western world. Luckily, though, their use is declining as more is being discovered about our gut microbiome and the importance of its ability to diversify and populate our GI tract in the first few years of life. Even brief antibiotic treatment can have long-term effects on microbiota composition, which may promote the development of disease (Lange *et al.* 2016).

The first exposure to antibiotics can occur during labor, when the mother tests positive for Group B *Streptococcus* (GBS) during routine screening and is given antibiotics to prevent transmission of the bacteria to the baby during labor. About one in every three or four women tests positive for GBS. GBS transmission in newborns can cause infections such as meningitis, pneumonia, or sepsis, which can be life-threatening, and the antibiotics are used as a prophylaxis. Research indicates that there is a delay in the microbial development up to 12 weeks of age with GBS antibiotic treatment, and the long-term effects are not yet fully understood (Stearns *et al.* 2017).

If babies are born prematurely (before 37 weeks gestation), they are nearly all given antibiotics in the Neonatal Intensive Care Unit (NICU) because they are vulnerable to infection. The antibiotic exposure, plus the fact that they are most often fed more formula than breast milk and have less physical contact with their mothers, creates prime conditions for microbial dysbiosis. It is known that premature babies are more likely to have chronic health issues such as asthma, eczema, higher rates of infections, dental, or behavioral and psychological problems. Stunted growth by age four was seen in premature babies with the most abnormal microbiome (University of South Florida 2019). Due to the potentially life-altering effects this can have for a child, any intervention that can improve outcomes is to be heralded. One such intervention showed benefits to the microbiota for premature babies when given *Bifidobacterium* and *Lactobacillus* as supplements; the babies' GI environment more closely resembled the normal environment of a full-term infant (Chelimo *et al.* 2020). This research was observational and is in its infancy, but given the promising results, offers hope that by harmonizing the microbial environment, many of these negative health conditions can be averted.

Repeated antibiotic exposure from birth up until the age of four was found to increase the likelihood of a child being overweight or obese by the age of four-and-a-half (Chelimo *et al.* 2020). Often what happens is that an initial bout of antibiotics disrupts the microbiota, leading to more illness, which then requires another dose of antibiotics, starting the damaging "antibiotic merry-go-round." This merry-go-round can begin so easily; my daughter had a viral cough one year which lingered for some time, so I took her to a walk-in clinic to have her checked out and to rule out anything more serious. The doctor checked her ears and noticed a little bit of redness and inflammation (my daughter had not complained of an earache). The doctor prescribed antibiotics to help clear the inflammation, but I knew in this case it was unnecessary and did not fill the prescription. My daughter recovered one hundred percent without the antibiotics, and I am fortunate that in her seven years of life she has never required them. It may have been a different story had I started with that first round.

Awareness surrounding the negative consequences of antibiotics has grown and doctors have made efforts to avoid prescribing them to young children unless absolutely necessary. Thanks to reduced antibiotic use, researchers from the BC Children's Hospital, the BC Center for Disease Control (BCCDC), and the University of British Columbia have found that the rates of pediatric asthma have also declined (Patrick *et al.* 2020). Their study analyzed data from about 225,000 children up to age four in British Columbia every year between 2000 and 2015, and from 2644 children in Vancouver, Edmonton, Winnipeg, and Toronto who are participants in the ongoing Canadian Healthy Infant Longitudinal Development (CHILD) cohort, which began in 2008 to study the development of various conditions from birth, including asthma, allergies, and obesity. Back in 2000, 70 percent of the children had received at least one course of antibiotics in their first year of life. By 2014, that number had dropped by half; most of the prescriptions in the early years had been for conditions such as viruses or colds, where there is no benefit and symptoms eventually resolve on their own. They found the rates of asthma increased by 24 percent with each 10 percent increase in antibiotic prescribing, and that it doubled the risk of asthma by age five if the prescription was in the first year of life. "Good bacteria play a vital role in childhood health and development. As this research shows, nurturing a diverse and robust microbiome, including the prudent use of antibiotics, can play a key role in the healthy development of a child's immune system and lead to life-long benefits," said Dr B. Brett Finlay, a professor in the University of British Columbia's Faculty of Medicine's Department of Biochemistry and Molecular Biology, and co-author of the study.[1]

Introducing solid foods too early

The WHO's recommendations for introducing solid foods for infants is at six months of age, with continued breastfeeding. Introducing solid foods too early could contribute to future health risks due to the negative changes observed in gut bacteria (Differding *et al.* 2020). Early introduction of solids before four months of age altered the gut microbiota in infants and was shown to increase their body mass index (BMI) by age five (Differding *et al.* 2020). Delaying solid foods plays a role in the healthy development of the gut microbiome, and is another aspect of the infant gut microbial health foundation.

Positive effects on the infant gut microbiome:

- Breastfeeding exclusively for the first six months of life.
- Vaginal birth.
- Avoiding unnecessary antibiotics.
- Living near green space.
- Having a pet in the home.
- Probiotic- and prebiotic-rich foods.

---

1   See www.bccdc.ca/about/news-stories/news-releases/2020/falling-childhood-asthma-rates-linked-to-declining-use-of-unnecessary-antibiotics

- Fiber found in fruit, vegetables and legumes, whole grains, and nuts.
- Diversity in the diet.
- Premature babies supplemented with *Bifidobacterium* and *Lactobacillus.*

Negative effects on the infant gut microbiome:

- C-section birth.
- Premature birth.
- Early and repeated antibiotic exposure.
- Early (before the age of four months) introduction to solid foods.
- Infant formula feeding due to lack of human milk oligosaccharides.

Our current understanding of the infant gut microbiome is that it is extremely important in the future health of the child. Looking at all the factors involved in the "seeding of the gut" as strengthening or as deleterious to the Spleen and Stomach network will help to broaden our treatment methods to incorporate the above recommendations as preventative and health-inducing measures.

CHAPTER 5

Spring

Spring means new beginnings and getting rid of the old to make way for the new, a season of true revitalization. Spring is the pivotal season of *Yin* transforming into *Yang*; day by day, *Yang* is increasing into the full *Yang* energy of summer. *Yin* elements of winter are still lingering, with the occasional spring snowfall and windy, cool temperatures, balanced by the upsurge of *Yang* as days become warmer, sunnier, and longer. *Yang* is seen bursting through the *Yin* unable to contain itself. The leaves are bursting out of the tree buds in which they have remained dormant all winter; seeds are germinating, breaking free from their *Yin* shells; and flowers and trees are blossoming, their fragrant scent carried along the breeze, letting us all know that the time of dormancy is complete.

Spring corresponds to the Wood element, which represents the Liver and Gallbladder organs. The Liver and Gallbladder share an interior–exterior relationship. In relation to the digestive system, the Liver sends bile to the Gallbladder to be stored until needed to emulsify fat, and they both depend on each other for the smooth flow of *Qi*. This is a strange relationship, as normally *Yin* organs store substances and *Yang* organs allow substances in and out. With the Liver and Gallbladder, this is reversed as the Liver is sending the bile to the Gallbladder for storage. When the Liver stagnates, the flow of bile is impaired and can cause digestive issues such as acid reflux, bloating, flatulence, indigestion, and constipation. This unsmooth flow of *Qi* can begin or worsens in the springtime—if the stagnation already exists—due to the energy moving into these organs. An imbalance in Liver *Qi*'s main etiology is repressed anger, frustration, or resentment, which causes circulation to become impaired. For children, Liver *Qi* stagnation is not usually seen until they are teenagers; they are excellent at immediately expressing their anger or frustration and, once out, forgotten about. They also do not drink alcohol or coffee, smoke, or take lots of prescription drugs, all of which, in excess, leads to stagnation. Most often, signs that would point to Liver *Qi* stagnation in adults—constipation, nausea, diarrhea, stomach pain, poor appetite, bloating—in children would instead be due to their immature developing organs, Spleen *Qi* deficiency, or food becoming stagnant leading to accumulation disorder.

The Wood element is attributed to the color green, which is apt for this time of the year; most of what is sprouting out of the ground is green, along with the green buds on trees and plants. It is a favorite season for many, waking up to the birds chirping, seeing the multitude of colors everywhere as flowers bloom, and getting back into the garden to start another year of harvest. This is a great opportunity for parents to include children in the gardening process, playing with dirt, planting seeds, deciding what vegetables or flowers to include, and helping in any way that is appropriate for their age. They will be more likely to eat their vegetables knowing that they played a part in their production. I remember reading about a dad who told his children not to eat anything out of the garden—a perfect way to make sure they do! Conversations with children about what grows in which season and what can be planted locally and seasonally will plant the seeds of healthful eating.

Busy lives and eating on the run may push children out of the kitchen. Encouraging parents to include children in the cooking process, to see foods before they are cooked, to visit local farms throughout the season, to have them pick out produce they think looks interesting and cook it up together, to quiz them on the names of vegetables at the grocery store, to buy them their own cookbook—these will all foster a connection to healthy food. Eating habits developed in infancy will influence eating habits in later years and adulthood (Grimm *et al.* 2014; University of Calgary 2009).

The best way to stay in harmony with the season of upward and outward expansion is to follow suit with increased movement and stretching. In *The Yellow Emperor's Classic of Medicine*, Huang Di states: "during this season it is advisable to retire early. Arise early also and go walking in order to absorb the fresh, invigorating energy. Since this is the season in which the universal energy begins anew and rejuvenates, one should attempt to correspond to it directly by being open and unsuppressed, both physically and emotionally" (Maoshing Ni 1995). It is still important at this time of year—as with autumn and winter—for children to have an early bedtime. Walking children to school, if possible, or parking a short distance away to allow for a walk will give them a chance to absorb the fresh air and feel energized before sitting in the classroom. Find ways in which to allow outdoor movement—this will be especially helpful for children who have trouble focusing at school.

The next guidance, as laid out in *The Yellow Emperor's Classic of Medicine*, is to allow all emotions to flow freely, parents and children alike. The emotions associated with the Liver are anger and frustration. There are many helpful resources available online and informative books for parents interested in how to teach children emotional regulation. This is a skill many adults were not given the opportunity to learn as children, and as such it can become a learning experience for the whole family.[1] Emotions are a natural part of being human, and the more we can feel them, the easier they are to manage. Identifying and naming an emotion is a skill most optimally learned in childhood. Suppressing emotions pushes the emotional blockage into the organs, and, as we age, creates health problems.

A paper published in 2019 looked at research done that establishes the link between emotional suppression and physiological consequences, including IBS, abdominal pain, indigestion, and headaches (Patel and Patel 2019). They also linked some of the longer-term health problems such as cancer and heart disease to emotional suppression. This is a well-understood concept in TCM, and acupuncture is a wonderful tool that allows these stuck emotions to be released from the affected organs. The most effective and preventative method is to identify and feel these emotions immediately, and not allow the stagnation to take root. Children are like little sponges— by recognizing and accepting from a young age that anger and frustration are normal parts of our everyday existence, they are set on the path of emotional intelligence. Allowing children to recognize this emotion as it comes up while discouraging actions such as hitting and lashing out will allow them to know that they have a right to be angry. This paves the way for a child who is comfortable with their feelings and can manage their anger constructively. As Aristotle once said, "Anybody can become angry—that is easy, but to be angry with the right person and to the right degree and at the right time and for the right purpose, and in the right way—that is not within everybody's power and is not easy."

Although this mindfulness towards emotions is a year-round consideration, spring is an opportune time to bring it up in the clinic to discuss with parents as it coincides so nicely with new beginnings and fresh starts and, of course, the connection to the Liver.

---

1   Aha!Parenting.com is one such site that offers great information, guidance, and book suggestions.

Spring meals

The energy of spring is about rising and moving outwards, and for this reason the pungent flavor is beneficial. This includes herbs and spices such as basil, bay leaves, rosemary, marjoram, thyme, ginger, and foods such as cabbage and onions. The pungent flavor is great at resolving stagnation as it promotes upward energy movement and increases Blood circulation. This aligns the energy in the body with the outside world. Children's energies naturally rise—due to their *Yang* nature—so *too much* pungency in the diet is not recommended. This is not usually a problem for children as they prefer sweet and salty anyway! The sweet flavor in foods such as carrots, sweet potatoes, beans, nuts, and seeds is also indicated as it harmonizes and softens the Liver, helping to ease tension, and acts as an analgesic. The sour flavor found in lemons, limes, and vinegar is helpful in the spring due to it being "most active in the Liver, where it counteracts the effects of rich, greasy food, functioning as a solvent and breaking down fats and protein" (Pitchford 2002, p.312). As the Wood element is nourished by the color green, all greens will benefit the Liver. It is quite common for children to receive green smoothies filled with kale, spinach, or any other greens on hand as it is thought this is a healthy and easy way for them to have it included in their diets. A green smoothie is difficult to digest, though, and will weaken Spleen *Qi* over time, so I don't recommend regular consumption for children. Steaming or sautéing greens will help to break down their tough, fibrous structures.

Sprouts such as mung beans and alfalfa are optimal at this time of year. They are not recommended for children under the age of five, though, due to the potential for harmful bacteria such as salmonella and *E. coli*. The long, slow-cooked meals of winter can start to give way to less cooking time. Cook vegetables on a high heat with oil for a short time so that the vegetable fibers are broken down slightly but there is still a crunch to them. Steam greens and vegetables or cook them in a little bit of water for a short duration. A little bit more raw food can be added into the diet again, as the weather starts to warm.

Food recommendations
Fruit

- Apples
- Blueberries
- Kiwifruit
- Strawberries.

Vegetables

- Arugula
- Asparagus
- Beets
- Bok choy
- Cabbage
- Carrots
- Celery
- Cucumber
- Chard
- Leeks
- Lettuce
- Mushrooms
- Onions
- Parsnips
- Potatoes
- Radishes
- Rhubarb
- Spinach
- Sweet potatoes
- Yams.

Beans and pulses

- Adzuki beans
- Black beans
- Black-eyed peas
- Butter (lima) beans
- Cannellini beans
- Chickpeas (garbanzo beans)
- Fava beans
- Great northern beans
- Kidney beans
- Lentils
- Lima beans
- Navy beans
- Peanuts
- Pinto beans
- Split peas (yellow and green)
- Tofu.

Grains

- Amaranth
- Barley
- Buckwheat
- Millet
- Oats
- Quinoa
- Rice
- Rye
- Spelt
- Teff
- Wheat (organic).

Nuts

Keep nuts and nut butters to a minimum.

- Almonds
- Brazil nuts
- Cashews
- Chestnuts
- Hazelnuts
- Pistachios
- Walnuts.

Seeds

- Chia seeds
- Flax seeds
- Hemp seeds
- Poppy seeds
- Pumpkin seeds
- Sesame seeds (black or white)
- Sunflower seeds.

Herbs and spices

PUNGENT SPICES

- Allspice
- Basil
- Bay leaf
- Black pepper
- Caraway seeds
- Cardamom
- Chive
- Cinnamon
- Cloves
- Coriander
- Cumin
- Curry
- Dill
- Fennel
- Fenugreek
- Ginger
- Marjoram
- Mustard seeds
- Nutmeg
- Thyme
- Sage
- Savory
- Star anise
- Thyme
- Turmeric.

OTHER SPICES

- Oregano
- Paprika
- Parsley leaf
- Vanilla.

Meat

- Beef
- Bison
- Chicken
- Chicken eggs
- Goat
- Pork
- Turkey.

Seafood

Locally harvested, fresh, and sustainable is recommended and will vary depending on geographical location.

- Anchovies
- Cod
- Crab
- Halibut
- Herring
- Lobster
- Mussels
- Prawns
- Salmon
- Sardines
- Scallops
- Shrimp

- Snapper
- Sole
- Trout
- Tuna
- Whitefish.

Breakfast ideas

Warm, nourishing breakfasts are beneficial year-round. As fruit starts to ripen, there will be more availability for fresh fruit to be eaten and added into breakfast porridges or granola. Opt for more seeds at this time of the year and less nuts.

- Bircher Müesli (see page 171)
- Buttermilk Pancakes (see page 172)
- Millet Muesli (see page 173)
- Scrambled Tofu (see page 175)
- Simple Granola (see page 176).

School lunch and snack ideas

- Apple Muffins (see page 178)
- Applesauce, with a pinch of cinnamon
- Black Bean Brownies (see page 178)
- Bliss Seed Balls (see page 179)
- Carrots, lightly cooked
- Chicken-fried rice with a type of bean and quick sautéed spring vegetables that the child enjoys
- Crackers (Homemade), topped with cheese or jam (see page 180)
- Dried fruit
- Hummus (see page 181)
- Kale Sunflower Chips (see page 182)
- Oat and Cardamom Muffins (see page 183)
- Oatmeal and Sesame Chocolate Chip Cookies (see page 184)
- Organic macaroni and cheese
- Pear Juice (see page 185)
- Peas (Side Dish) (see page 202)
- Pickles
- Popcorn (Homemade), sprinkled with nutritional yeast or cinnamon (see page 186)
- Puffed Amaranth and Seed Bar (see page 187)

- Roasted Chickpeas (see page 188)
- Sliced apple, rubbed with a little lemon juice
- Smoked salmon
- Spinach and Chive Muffins (see page 189)
- Stewed Apple and Pear (see page 190)
- Tuna sandwich
- Whole grain or gluten-free wrap with beans, cheese, spinach, rice, and a little yoghurt as the sauce.

Home lunch and dinner ideas

- Anellini Pasta with Broccoli and Ham (see page 192)
- Cabbage, the German Way (see page 193)
- Carrot Salad (see page 194)
- Honey and Ginger Wild Salmon (see page 196)
- Leek and Potato Soup (see page 197)
- Lentil Dal (see page 198)
- Millet (Side Dish) (see page 199)
- Millet Salad (see page 199)
- Millet Soupy Porridge (see page 200)
- Orange Chicken (or Tofu) and Almonds (see page 201)
- Peas (Side Dish) (see page 202)
- Pesto d'Urtica (see page 203)
- Vegetarian lasagna (see page 206).

CHAPTER 6

Summer

A truly abundant, life-giving, energizing season, summer is the utmost *Yang* time of year and the longer, hotter, sunnier days are a child's dream. Produce, plants, and trees are growing rapidly, and the farmers' markets abound with fresh vegetables and ripe fruit. Summer feels as if it unfolds over a long expanse of unstructured, play-filled, never-ending time of pure joy, laughter, and fun. Around us the world is alive, and the *Yang* energy of the sun infuses brightness and life into our being. We feel the pull to be outdoors, interacting with others; picnics, al fresco dining, and roasting food over a campfire are quintessential summer enjoyment.

Summer corresponds to the Fire element, which represents the organs of the Heart and Small Intestine. The Heart and Small Intestine share an interior–exterior relationship. The Heart is reliant on the organs for nourishment, unlike the Spleen, which *delivers* postnatal *Qi* to all the organs. The Heart is metaphorically regarded as the monarch and requires clear thinking to make decisions for the kingdom, the other organs. Therefore, the organs will give of themselves to make sure the Heart is taken care of. The spirit, or *Shen*, as it is called in TCM, corresponds to but has a much greater meaning than the English word "mind," and is housed in the Heart. A healthy *Shen* emanates from the Heart as light that shines from the behind the eyes, mental acuity, and a calm mind. When the Heart is not in balance, issues with sleep, anxiety, mental restlessness, and hyperactivity can be seen in children. It is with the Heart that we can realize the importance of a healthy digestive system; a harmonious Spleen, as discussed in Chapter 2, will have the energy to nourish all the systems and the organs will in turn nourish the Heart. As Giovanni Maciocia states in *The Foundations of Chinese Medicine*, "If the Heart is strong and Blood abundant, there will be normal mental activity, a balanced emotional life, a clear consciousness, a good memory, keen thinking and good sleep. If the Heart is weak and

Blood deficient there may be mental problems (such as depression), poor memory, dull thinking, insomnia, or somnolence and in extreme cases, unconsciousness" (1989, p.72).

The connection of digestive health to the emotions has become a well-researched field. The gut–brain axis is the complex system of communication between the central nervous system (brain and spinal cord) and the gastrointestinal (GI) tract. The GI tract is home to the largest concentration and highest diversity of bacterial species called the microbiome. How these bacteria and the individual colonies that we each have influence our being is an area of continued study. What is clear is that there is a connection between cognitive ability, depression, anxiety, and gut health (Valles-Colomer *et al.* 2019). Interestingly, recent research has found a link between dysbiosis (microbial imbalance) and cardiovascular disease (Jin *et al.* 2019). This has led to allopathic medicine using optimization of diet and the use of probiotics for treatment of heart disease. TCM has understood this for millennia—when the gut is not happy, the Heart/Mind is unsettled.

Although the Heart does not play a direct role in digestion or elimination, its paired organ, the Small Intestine, does. Most of the absorption of nutrients and minerals from food takes place here and is sent to the Spleen to be distributed to the rest of the body. The Small Intestine has the function of separating the pure from the turbid, both with foodstuff and our thoughts. The pure is sent to the Spleen for distribution and the impure is sent to the Large Intestine for elimination in the stools and to the Bladder to form urine. The Spleen also plays an important role in the digestion process here. If the Spleen is weak and has not pre-digested the food properly, then the Small Intestine will have extra work to do to make up for it. This may cause a problem in separating the pure from the turbid. Some symptoms that might arise in children from this turbidity include:

- Loose stools.
- Lower abdominal pain.
- Borborygmus.
- Trouble deciphering between right and wrong (up until about age five it is up to the parent or guardian to teach children what is right and wrong). This example applies to older children who have trouble making the distinction. For example, most school-age children would know it is not right to take toys home from school; with a Small Intestine imbalance, this may not be clear to the child who has a habit of taking things home that do not belong to them.

The emotion of joy nourishes the Heart. The true enjoyment of meals and eating helps in the alchemical transformation of food into *Qi*; in the Five Element generating cycle the Heart/Fire is the mother of the Spleen/Earth. The Heart is also nourished through connection to family and friends (love) and gratitude for the food.

Summer meals

Children are more prone to heat illness than adults, due to their smaller size, weighing less, and having a larger relative surface area than adults. Pound for pound, children accumulate more heat than adults during an activity such as cycling or walking, and they sweat less. Therefore, it is important to increase the intake of *Yin* cooling foods to offset the *Yang* heating nature of summer. These foods will help to cool and moisten the body and to replenish the fluids lost through sweat. Because children have an immature Spleen and Stomach, it is necessary to balance the amount of cooling or cold foods with warming foods to protect their digestive energy. Foods such as cucumber, lettuce, and watermelon are very cooling and have a high water content. An increase in raw food is recommended in the summer, but with children this would need to be watched carefully depending on their individual digestive fire. If there is an increase in loose stools or diarrhea that is not connected to illness, this would indicate too much raw and cold food that is not being digested properly.

Cooking vegetables quickly at a high heat or steaming them for a short time are both great summer methods to soften vegetables without overcooking. The flavor associated with the Heart is bitter. Bitter has the action of clearing heat, detoxifying, and drying dampness. You can be certain that anything ingested with a bitter flavor will be healthy for the body. Bitter flavor can be tasted in foods such as rye, kale, arugula, eggplants (aubergines), chicory, dark chocolate, and endives. Children have about thirty thousand taste buds spread throughout their mouth, and by the time they are adults, only about a third of these remain. Due to this fact, the bitter flavor is heightened in children. There is a reason why infants reject the bitter flavor—many poisonous plants are bitter, and this is a life-saving, inborn, unlearned response (Mennella and Bobowski 2015). Bitter is not appreciated until the adolescent years unless it is masked by a little sweetness. Parents can be reassured not to sweat it when their little ones will not touch certain bitter foods. I still recommend adding a little to their plates so they can see the adult eating it and become comfortable with seeing it and possibly tasting (or licking) it here and there.

Foods with pungency, such as ginger, black pepper, and cinnamon bark, are helpful in the summer as they have an outward movement to promote sweating. Therefore, cuisine in hot countries is often very spicy; the spices induce sweating, which cools the body. If too much greasy, heavy food is eaten, this will instead cause lethargy and indigestion. This includes damp-forming foods such as sugar and milk combinations (ice cream, chocolate milk), sugar and flour combinations (pastries, many packaged snacks), an excess of nuts, too many eggs, and deep-fried foods. Hotter days usually equal a smaller appetite; sticking to lighter fare such as salads, fish, fruits, and rice will be easy on the digestion. In TCM it is common to serve soups made with cooling and sour ingredients (mung beans, watermelon, tomatoes) to increase fluids, boost hydration, and clear heat. Mung beans are traditionally eaten in the summer to help clear summer heat and prevent heat stroke. It is also the season to enjoy the vast variety and amount of fresh fruit available; most fruit is cooling and hydrating. Herbs such as mint, lemon balm, chrysanthemum, and raspberry leaf are cooling and can be brewed into delicious teas. The color associated with Fire is (not surprisingly) red. Red is a very vibrant, dynamic, warming color, and therefore aptly connected with the summer and the *Yang* time of the year. All red foods will help to nourish the Heart: cherries, strawberries, raspberries, watermelon, red peppers, beets, and goji berries are a few.

Cold foods like ice cream, popsicles, and iced drinks are commonly consumed in the summer with the idea that they refresh and cool children down. As Paul Pitchford states in *Healing with Whole Foods*, "Coldness causes contraction; it holds in sweat and heat and interferes with digestion. Iced drinks and ice cream actually contract the stomach and stop digestion" (2002, p.331). Sweating and the process of evaporation off the skin is an important mechanism used for thermoregulation in the body, and is best supported by loose, breathable clothing and, counter-intuitively, hot or warm drinks. Cold food and drink can seem refreshing and perfect for keeping children cool in the summer, but research done at the University of Ottawa's School of Human Kinetics showed that a hot beverage cools us down better. When a hot drink is consumed on a hot day and the sweat can evaporate (and the person isn't bundled up), the body cools down (Bain, Lesperance, and Jay 2012).

The longer days of summer allow for less sleep. Staying up later while still getting up early will not leave children bleary eyed as it would in the colder months of the year. As a parent, I have learned over time that this is a time of year to "go with the flow" and to try not to resist the natural rhythm. Trying to get children into bed early when it is hot and bright outside goes against this rhythm and can create strife.

Many wonderful memories are created for children over the summer months, especially as, for many, this is their school holiday time. Meals taken outdoors can be enjoyed in the shade of a tree, sitting at a picnic table, or on a blanket by a lake.

Food recommendations
Fruit
Seasonal to the local geographical area.

- Apples
- Apricots
- Avocados
- Blueberries
- Blackberries
- Boysenberries
- Cherries
- Figs

- Grapes
- Loganberries
- Mandarins
- Melon
- Nectarines
- Oranges
- Peaches
- Plums

- Raspberries
- Rhubarb
- Strawberries
- Tayberries
- Tomatoes
- Watermelon.

Vegetables

- Arugula
- Asparagus
- Bell peppers, green—cooling
- Bell peppers, red, orange, and yellow—neutral
- Beans
- Beets

- Bok choy
- Carrots
- Cherry tomatoes
- Corn
- Cucumber
- Eggplants (aubergines)
- Lettuce
- Peas

- Potatoes
- Radishes
- Spinach
- Sugar snap peas
- Tomatoes
- Yellow squash
- Zucchini (courgettes).

Beans and pulses

- Adzuki beans
- Black beans
- Black-eyed peas

- Butter (lima) beans
- Cannellini beans

- Chickpeas (garbanzo beans)
- Fava beans

- Great northern beans
- Kidney beans
- Lentils
- Lima beans
- Miso
- Mung beans (very cooling, small amounts only)
- Navy beans
- Peanuts
- Pinto beans
- Split peas (yellow and green)
- Tofu.

Grains

- Amaranth
- Barley
- Buckwheat
- Millet
- Oats
- Quinoa
- Rice
- Rye
- Spelt
- Teff
- Wheat (organic).

Seeds

- Chia seeds
- Flax seeds
- Hemp seeds
- Poppy seeds
- Pumpkin seeds
- Sesame seeds (black or white)
- Sunflower seeds.

Herbs and spices

COOLING HERBS AND SPICES

- Chrysanthemum
- Cilantro (coriander)
- Mint
- Spearmint.

OTHER HERBS AND SPICES

- Basil
- Black pepper
- Caraway seeds
- Cardamom
- Cinnamon
- Coriander
- Cumin
- Curry
- Dill
- Fennel
- Fenugreek
- Ginger
- Marjoram
- Mustard seeds
- Nutmeg
- Oregano
- Paprika
- Parsley leaf
- Sage
- Savory
- Thyme
- Turmeric
- Vanilla.

Meat

- Beef
- Bison
- Chicken
- Chicken eggs
- Goat
- Pork
- Turkey.

Seafood

Locally harvested, fresh, and sustainable is recommended and will vary depending on geographical location.

- Anchovies
- Bluefish
- Clams
- Cod
- Crab
- Halibut
- Herring
- Lobster
- Mackerel
- Mussels
- Prawns
- Salmon
- Sardines
- Scallops
- Shrimp
- Snapper
- Sole
- Trout
- Tuna
- Whitefish.

Breakfast ideas

Warm, nourishing breakfasts are beneficial year-round. Summer fruit is abundant, and this is the time of year to enjoy it as much as possible! Eat mainly seeds throughout the hotter months of the year.

- Bircher Müesli (see page 171)
- Buttermilk Pancakes (see page 172)
- Millet Muesli (see page 173)
- Scrambled Tofu (see page 175)
- Simple Granola (see page 176)
- Summer Mung Bean Breakfast Soup (see page 177).

School lunch and snack ideas

- Apple Muffins (see page 178)
- Applesauce, with a pinch of cinnamon
- Berries
- Black Bean Brownies (see page 178)
- Bliss Seed Balls (see page 179)
- Cabbage, the German Way (see page 193)

- Cherry tomatoes
- Chicken-fried rice with a type of bean and quick sautéed spring vegetables that the child enjoys
- Crackers (Homemade), topped with cheese or jam (see page 180)
- Cucumber Salad (see page 181)
- Dried fruit
- Hummus (see page 181)
- Kale Sunflower Chips (see page 182)
- Oatmeal and Sesame Chocolate Chip Cookies (see page 184)
- Oranges
- Organic macaroni and cheese
- Pear Juice (see page 185)
- Peas (Side Dish) (see page 202)
- Pickles
- Popcorn (Homemade), sprinkled with nutritional yeast or cinnamon (see page 186)
- Puffed Amaranth and Seed Bar (see page 187)
- Roasted Chickpeas (see page 188)
- Sliced apples, rubbed with a little lemon juice
- Smoked salmon
- Spinach and Chive Muffins (see page 189)
- Stewed Apple and Pear (see page 190)
- Tuna sandwich
- Veggies, raw, seasonal, such as snap peas, carrots, cucumber, peppers, beans, radishes
- Whole grain or gluten-free wrap with beans, cheese, sautéed seasonal veggies, rice, and yoghurt sauce to spread.

Home lunch and dinner ideas

- Anellini Pasta with Broccoli and Ham (see page 192)
- Cabbage, the German Way (see page 193)
- Carrot Salad (see page 194)
- Honey and Ginger Wild Salmon (see page 196)
- Lentil Dal (see page 198)
- Millet (Side Dish) (see page 199)
- Millet Salad (see page 199)
- Millet Soupy Porridge (see page 200)

- Orange Chicken (or Tofu) and Almonds (see page 201)
- Peas (Side Dish) (see page 202)
- Vegetarian Lasagna (see page 206)
- Watermelon and Feta Summer Salad (see page 207).

CHAPTER 7

Autumn

The essence of food is received through the sense of smell, which is related to the Metal Element and lungs. The appetite is stimulated by the warm fragrance of baked and sautéed food—concentrated foods and roots thicken the blood for cooler weather.

Pitchford (2002, p.347)

Autumn heralds new beginnings for children. This time of the year is busy and can feel more like the mark of a new year than the January 1st calendar New Year. School gets under way, extracurricular programs commence, and the long, lazy, unstructured days of summer flow back into day-to-day routines. There is a shift from the expansive qualities of summer (playing outdoors late into the day, requiring less sleep, and feeling energized by the sun's rays) to the contracting properties of autumn (gathering together, turning inwards, and spending a little less time outdoors). There is a veritable abundance of crop harvests and magnificent color changes—this is truly a time when we can attest to the wonders of Mother Nature. Shades of red, orange, gold, brown, and green grace the landscape, and the same wondrous color assortment overflows in the produce bins at markets and stores. Piles of crispy leaves are an irresistible delight for children! The air begins to turn crisp and cool with an accompanying dryness, and the *Yin* darkness starts to encroach on the *Yang* light.

Autumn is the transition period from *Yang* summer to *Yin* winter. This season corresponds to the Metal element, which represents the organs of the Lung and Large Intestine. The Lung and Large Intestine share an interior–exterior connection. The Lungs are responsible for taking in (breathing in air for oxygen) while the Large Intestine is responsible for elimination (getting rid of waste and whatever else the body no longer needs). Both the aspects of "taking in" and "eliminating" are occurring in nature this season. *Harvest* was the earliest name for autumn, and indicates this is the season for gathering and harvesting all the produce that has grown through the summer. Autumn is also quintessential to "letting go"—trees shed their leaves, plants cast their seeds to the wind, gardens release their harvest of the season, and many insects and animals migrate deeper into the ground or move south as the cold weather approaches. In the same sense, the Large Intestine's function is also one of "letting go," the elimination process of what no longer serves the body. Children can occasionally have issues with constipation when they are having trouble letting go of something in their lives; they might be afraid of letting go of a loved one for the day when starting daycare or preschool, or believe their stool to be a part of themselves and resist or fear letting go of this into the toilet.

The Lungs in children are immature; adults have around 300 million air sacs, whereas, at birth, babies have around 20–50 million. New air sacs continue to develop in children until the teenage years, at which point they are fully developed. The Lungs control the circulation of Defensive *Qi* (*Wei Qi*) throughout the body, which circulates in the exterior through the skin and flesh, its main function to help prevent the invasion of external pathogenic factors (that is, Wind, Cold, Heat, and Damp). These external pathogenic factors can manifest as different illnesses (such as colds, flu, or a cough) if they are able to penetrate the body through Defensive *Qi*. Well-functioning Defensive *Qi* is likened to a robust immune system. Children's Defensive *Qi* is immature until around age seven or eight, and can be more easily invaded until then; for this reason, small children are particularly susceptible to frequent colds or flu that are starting to circulate at this time of year. Food *Qi* produced by the Spleen and Stomach nourishes Defensive *Qi* that underpins the support of a nourishing diet to a well-balanced immune response.

Autumn is that in-between time when temperatures can fluctuate and become very cold as soon as the sun hides behind a cloud or the wind picks up. Vests are a practical item of clothing for children in the fall; their chests are covered front and back, keeping their delicate Lung area warm. Vests prevent overheating and children are less likely to fling them off. The heightened activity of summer can now start to wind down with this pivotal transition time from *Yang* to *Yin*. The later bedtimes of summer should shift earlier, and it is a time to "gather one's spirit and energy" (Maoshing Ni 1995, p.6). For children this means set routines in which they aren't overscheduled, protecting their chest and upper back area from the wind and cold, and eating the right seasonal foods.

Autumn meals

Meals should start to reflect the cooler days of autumn. This entails transitioning into eating more warming meals that have been cooked for a little longer at a lower temperature. Raw vegetables and fruit consumption can start to decrease. For children, daily dried fruit in their diets helps with fiber intake, along with the benefits of fruit without the cooling qualities of too much fresh fruit. The inclusion of warming spices will raise the thermal nature of dishes and enhance digestion. Cold, raw salads (such as green salads, Greek salad, and Caesar salad) should be kept to a minimum until the warmer days of summer return. The berries, stone fruit, and melons of summer are no longer available, and instead, apples, pears, and kiwifruit are the mainstays of the season. Images of roasted butternut soup, pumpkin pie, and roasted acorn squash are easily conjured when thinking of autumn. Winter squash and their natural sweetness and earthy, yellow tones are perfect for supplementing the Spleen and Stomach of children.

The flavor associated with the Lungs is pungent. Pungent foods are *Yang* and ascending, move up into the Lungs to clear and help keep the mucous flowing, preventing it from accumulating—children don't need a lot to reap the benefits! In fact, incorporating too much pungent food for children, especially in this dry season, can create internal dryness issues (such as constipation, dry skin, and dry throat) as pungency is drying. Pungent foods can be used at any time of the year to aid Lung conditions. Examples of pungent foods include garlic, ginger, chilies, peppers, onions, leeks, kale, mustard greens, and fennel. To help balance pungency, the sour flavor preserves fluids (*Yin*) in the body. The sour flavor is astringing, which perfectly parallels the contracting essence of autumn as our energies go inwards to conserve it through winter. Examples of sour foods include apples, sauerkraut, vinegars, lemons, limes, yoghurt, sourdough bread, and fermented dishes. White foods (apples, pears) are said to nourish the Lungs.

Moistening foods (listed below) can be included in the diet in areas where autumn brings dryness to the climate. Chapped lips and dry skin, nose, and throat are signs of dryness in the body.

Food recommendations
Fruit
Seasonal to the local geographical area.

- Apples
- Cranberries
- Figs

- Kiwifruit
- Local grapes
- Pears
- Persimmons
- Quince.

Vegetables

- Beets
- Broccoli
- Brussels sprouts
- Cabbage
- Carrots
- Cauliflower
- Celery
- Celery root
- Chard
- Cherry tomatoes
- Collard greens
- Curly endive
- Eggplants (aubergines)
- Fennel
- Kale
- Leeks
- Mushrooms (Shiitake is especially effective for strengthening the immune system)
- Onions
- Peppers
- Potatoes
- Pumpkin
- Sweet potatoes
- Tomatoes
- Winter squash (e.g. butternut, spaghetti, acorn, delicata, kabocha, red kuri, carnival, buttercup, hubbard, banana).

Beans and pulses
White beans especially.

- Adzuki beans
- Black beans
- Black-eyed peas
- Butter (lima) beans
- Cannellini beans
- Chickpeas (garbanzo beans)
- Fava beans
- Great northern beans
- Kidney beans
- Lentils
- Lima beans
- Navy beans
- Peanuts
- Pinto beans
- Split peas (yellow and green)
- Tofu.

Grains

- Amaranth
- Barley
- Buckwheat
- Millet
- Oats
- Quinoa
- Rice
- Rye
- Spelt
- Teff
- Wheat (organic).

Nuts

- Almonds
- Brazil nuts
- Chestnuts
- Hazelnuts
- Pecans
- Pine nuts
- Pistachios
- Walnuts.

Seeds

- Chia seeds
- Flax seeds
- Hemp seeds
- Poppy seeds
- Pumpkin seeds
- Sesame seeds (black or white)
- Sunflower seeds.

Herbs and spices

PUNGENT SPICES

- Allspice
- Basil
- Bay leaf
- Black pepper
- Caraway seeds
- Cardamom
- Cinnamon
- Cloves
- Coriander
- Cumin
- Curry
- Dill
- Fennel
- Fenugreek
- Ginger
- Marjoram
- Mustard seeds
- Nutmeg
- Sage
- Savory
- Star anise
- Thyme
- Turmeric.

OTHER SPICES

- Oregano
- Paprika
- Parsley leaf
- Vanilla.

Meat

- Beef
- Bison
- Chicken
- Chicken eggs
- Goat
- Lamb
- Pork
- Turkey.

Seafood

Locally harvested, fresh, and sustainable is recommended, and will vary depending on geographical location.

- Anchovies
- Herring
- Lobster
- Mussels
- Prawns
- Salmon
- Sardines
- Scallops
- Shrimp
- Snapper
- Sole
- Trout
- Tuna
- Whitefish.

Foods with moistening qualities

- Almonds
- Barley malt
- Clams
- Crab
- Eggs
- Goat's cheese
- Herring
- Honey
- Millet
- Peanuts
- Pine nuts
- Pistachios
- Pork
- Pumpkin
- Sesame oil
- Sesame seeds
- Tempeh
- Tofu.

Breakfast ideas

Warm, nourishing breakfasts are beneficial year-round. Winter squash is plentiful; squash and pumpkin puree can be added to pancakes or warmed up with muesli.

- Bircher Müesli (see page 171)
- Buttermilk Pancakes (see page 172)
- Millet Muesli (see page 173)
- Nut-Ella, spread on toast (see page 174)
- Scrambled Tofu (see page 175)
- Simple Granola (see page 176).

School lunch and snack ideas

- Apple Muffins (see page 178)
- Applesauce, with a pinch of cinnamon
- Black Bean Brownies (see page 178)
- Bliss Seed Balls (see page 179)
- Candied Ginger (see page 148)

- Chicken-fried rice with a type of bean and quick sautéed spring vegetables that the child enjoys
- Crackers (Homemade), topped with cheese or jam (see page 180)
- Dried fruit
- Hummus (see page 181)
- Kale Sunflower Chips (see pages 182)
- Oat and Cardamom Muffins (see page 183)
- Oatmeal and Sesame Chocolate Chip Cookies (see page 184)
- Organic macaroni and cheese
- Pear Juice (see page 185)
- Pear Smoothy (see page 186)
- Peas (Side Dish) (see page 202)
- Popcorn (Homemade), sprinkled with nutritional yeast or cinnamon (see page 186)
- Puffed Amaranth and Seed Bar (see page 187)
- Puffed Lotus Seed with Pumpkin Pie Spice (see page 122)
- Roasted Chickpeas (see page 188)
- Sliced apples, rubbed with a little lemon juice
- Smoked salmon
- Sweet Potato Toast (see page 189)
- Tuna sandwich
- Veggies—a little less raw and transitioning to more cooked veggies as the weather cools
- Whole grain or gluten-free wrap with beans, cheese, cooked seasonal veggies, rice, and yoghurt sauce to spread
- Winter Squash Loaf (see page 191).

Home lunch and dinner ideas

- Anellini Pasta with Broccoli and Ham (see page 192)
- Cabbage, the German Way (see page 193)
- Celeriac (Celery Root) Salad (see page 195)
- Crock Pot Beef and Bean, or only Bean, Chili (see page 195)
- Honey and Ginger Wild Salmon (see page 196)
- Leek and Potato Soup (see page 197)
- Lentil Dal (see page 198)
- Millet (Side Dish) (see page 199)
- Millet Soupy Porridge (see page 200)

- Orange Chicken (or Tofu) and Almonds (see page 201)
- Peas (Side Dish) (see page 202)
- Steamed Egg Soup (see page 204)
- Sweet Potato and Butter Bean (Lima Bean) Soup (see page 205)
- Vegetarian Lasagna (see page 206).

CHAPTER 8

Winter

The days of winter are darker, colder, and shorter; it is the most *Yin* time of the year. Many plants are dormant and observing nature and it can seem as if life is on pause—a sharp contrast from the active, hot, long, *Yang* days of summer. Icicles hang in mid-drip from the edges of homes, the fast, vigorous summer growth of plants and vegetables shifts to a snail's pace, and many animals have slowed their metabolisms and dug their winter dens to enter their hibernation or dormant period. In many places snow will blanket the ground, replacing the fallen foliage of autumn. Frost paints the ground and its surroundings an icy white. Various ponds and lakes freeze over, and the chill in the air reveals our breath. Bowls of steaming soup or chili offer comfort, and deeply warm the core of the body to the tips of the fingers and toes after time spent playing outdoors in the cold.

Winter corresponds to the Water element, which represents the organs of the Kidneys and Bladder and share an interior–exterior connection. The Kidneys store the Essence (*Jing*) and control the functions of birth, growth, and reproduction. The Bladder's function is to transform and excrete fluids and receive the *Qi* necessary for this function from the Kidneys. We see the connection between the Kidneys and Bladder in children who have issues with bedwetting (nocturnal enuresis). Fear is the emotion connected to the Kidneys; fear or worries in children can result in bedwetting as can a deficiency of the Kidney *Qi*. The salty flavor—the only flavor that is also a mineral—goes to the Kidneys.

The Kidneys provide the foundational energy responsible for growth and development. Kidney Essence (*Jing*) controls the growth of bones, teeth, hair, and brain development. Parents pass Essence (*Jing*) down to the fetus, which forms a child's pre-Heaven Essence (pre-Heaven *Jing*). This is the inherited constitutional makeup of an individual child's physical and mental baseline. This Essence is essentially non-renewable and can only be conserved by striving for balance in life. For children, this involves getting enough sleep, a nourishing diet, and not overdoing sports and exercise. If children develop a horizontal line (a little wrinkle) across the upper chin, it is a sign they are overscheduled, and overusing and tapping into their non-renewable essence. Post-Heaven Essence (post-Heaven *Jing*) *is* renewable, made from food and fluids, and is stored in the Kidneys. Giovanni Maciocia, author of *The Foundations of Chinese Medicine*, writes, "This is the essence which is refined and extracted from food and fluids by the Stomach and Spleen after birth. After birth, the baby starts eating, drinking, and breathing, its Lungs, Stomach and Spleen start functioning to produce *Qi* from food, drink and air" (1989, p.38). He goes on to write, "Because the Stomach and Spleen are responsible for the digestion of food and the transformation and transportation of food essences ultimately leading to the production of *Qi*, the Post-Heaven Essence is closely related to Stomach and Spleen" (1989, pp.38–39). Protecting and nourishing digestion is intricately connected to the production of essence and the strength of the Kidneys. Children are in a constant state of rapid growth and development; this therefore links back to the importance of a proper diet to ensure optimal development. Some examples of Kidney Essence deficiency in children are stunted growth and soft, weak bones and teeth.

As the days get even colder and darker, a *Yin* way of being will promote harmony in this season. *Yin* being means more rest time, longer sleeps (early to bed and later to rise), and less overall activity. It is especially important to keep the Middle Burner warmed with warming food and drink at this time of year, to balance the exterior cold. The lower back area, where the Kidneys are located, is sensitive to cold and must be kept covered to keep the Kidneys warm. The Gate of Vitality (Ming Men) is located in the lower back between the Kidneys, and provides the fire and heat for all the bodily functions, including aiding digestion by supplying warmth to the Spleen and Stomach. A heat pack for children's lower back area can take the edge off a chill and help stoke the Gate of Vitality's fire. The feet are also connected to the Kidneys through the bottom of the foot at the acupuncture point Kidney-1 (Gushing Spring). At home, wood or laminate floors are much colder than carpet, and investing in a warm pair of sheepskin or wool slippers will help benefit children's immune systems. Researchers at Cardiff University's Common Cold Centre have been studying colds and flus for over 30 years. One of their research studies involved acute chilling of the feet and the effects on the immune system. In the study, 180 volunteers were asked to soak their bare feet in icy water for 20 minutes. Researchers found that 29 percent of the volunteers developed a cold within five days, compared to only 9 percent in the control group. The explanation? When our feet become chilled, the blood vessels in the nasal passages constrict, effectively shutting off the warm blood that supplies the white cells, which fight infection (Johnson and Eccles 2005).

The battle to keep children bundled up is one common power struggle parents deal with when raising children. Children are *Yang* in nature and usually run warm—they don't feel the cold easily! This is especially obvious after recess or lunch playtime, when playgrounds are littered with forgotten coats, mitts, and hats! It helps to layer kids up with undershirts, long johns, wool sweaters, and socks. A child's-size haramaki, a piece of Japanese clothing worn around the waist to keep the core warm, can be used as an added layer of protection. This way, even if their coats come off, they are still well insulated. Merino wool is especially effective as a base layer, as it regulates body temperature and transports sweat away as vapor. Outdoor sports at this time of year can introduce cold (and dampness, depending on the climate) into the channels of the body. Repeated exposure without proper clothing protection can eventually turn into issues such as painful menstrual cramps, urination issues (pain, discomfort, or burning sensations), and injury to muscles, tendons, or ligaments.

Energetically, winter is a time to go inwards and to slow down. All around us nature is resting and guiding us to do the same. Just as grass, plants, and trees have a dormancy period, so we need to respect that it is a time of year to recharge batteries. Lazy weekends spent reading, doing puzzles and artwork, or engaging in unstructured play will do wonders for children's wellbeing and immunity. The holiday season, with the hustle and bustle of parties, concerts, and gatherings, is often an incredibly busy time of the year; plan and create space in the calendar for downtime, which will honor the season's need for rest and hibernation.

Children, being naturally *Yang* in nature, will still, of course, require exercise—staying bundled and getting them out to the park, woods, lake, or ocean will balance their need for movement and play.

Winter meals

The diet at this time of year should be mostly cooked, warming, and seasonally attuned. Raw vegetables and fresh fruit are too cold for the digestion and need to be a very minimal part of the diet in the winter months—not always an easy feat, as I know how much kids love their raw veggies! Any fruit eaten raw should be in season or of a variety that stores well through the winter, such as apples, pears, and kiwifruit. Occasionally, other cooked fruit—such as berries—can be incorporated for variety. Frozen blueberries or strawberries can be tossed into a pancake mixture or baked into muffins for a delightful treat. Cooking these fruits warms them up energetically.

Cooking methods that infuse a lot of heat into dishes consist of roasting, baking, and frying. Cooking foods longer, at lower temperatures, also incorporates warmth. Pressure cookers and Instant Pots are convenient for reducing cooking time while still ensuring food is cooked enough to acquire the level of heat that will warm the body and digestion. Spices such as cinnamon, nutmeg, cardamom, star anise, paprika, cloves, cumin, thyme, and sage help with flavoring and warm the *Yang*. Many popular winter dishes (dals, soups, chilis, stews, etc.) can disguise and up the intake of vegetables that are low on the palatable scale for children. Other ways of incorporating cooked vegetables are to bake squash or root vegetables into savory or sweet muffins and loaves, add them to omelets, or puree into sauces. However, it is also important for children to see, taste, smell, and feel the texture of vegetables, as it is only through continued exposure and familiarity that they can become comfortable with new foods.

Salty foods help to deliver the energetics of what we are eating to the Kidneys because of their down-bearing action. The salty flavor does supplement the Kidneys, but in our culture, which normalizes processed foods and eating out, it is important to pay attention and to limit how much salt finds its way into the diet. Excess salt intake can easily dehydrate children. Infants get salt in breast milk, and this is all they require. Infants from seven months to a year are recommended to have 0.4 grams of salt per day, children from one to eight years about 1 gram and ages 9–13 about 1.5 grams. To put this into perspective, 1 gram of salt is equal to ¼ of a teaspoon. One cup of canned chicken soup can contain 800 milligrams, which is almost the full daily allowance for a child. It is this flavor, along with sweet, that we need to be the most mindful of minimizing in children. An excess of salt weakens the Kidneys. Potato chips, processed foods, lunch and deli meats, sports drinks, and pizza are all known to be high in sodium.

A teaspoon of salt added to a pot of soup is all that is required to enable the energetics of the food to reach the Kidneys. Mineral-rich foods like seaweed, nuts, seeds, beans, mushrooms, bone broths, and dark leafy greens also deeply nourish the Kidneys. The color of the Kidneys is black, so any dark-colored or kidney-shaped foods also nourish the Kidneys.

Food recommendations
Fruit
Seasonal to the local geographical area, and/or fruit that stores well through the winter.

- Apples
- Kiwifruit
- Pears.

Vegetables
Root vegetables are especially nourishing in the winter.

ROOT VEGETABLES

- Beets
- Carrots
- Celery root
- Daikon
- Fennel
- Kohlrabi
- Parsnips
- Potatoes
- Rutabaga (swede)
- Sweet potatoes
- Turnips
- Yams.

OTHER VEGETABLES

- Broccoli
- Brussels sprouts
- Cabbage
- Cauliflower
- Chard
- Celery
- Collard greens
- Curly endive
- Eggplants (aubergines)
- Garlic
- Kale
- Leeks
- Mushrooms (Shiitake mushrooms are especially effective for strengthening the immune system)
- Onions
- Peppers
- Pumpkin
- Winter squash (e.g. butternut, spaghetti, acorn, delicata, kabocha, red kuri, carnival, buttercup, hubbard, banana, to name just a few).

Beans and pulses
The darker beans especially.

- Adzuki beans
- Black beans
- Black-eyed peas
- Butter (lima) beans
- Cannellini beans
- Chickpeas (garbanzo beans)
- Fava beans
- Great northern beans
- Kidney bean
- Lentils
- Lima beans

- Miso
- Navy beans
- Peanuts
- Pinto beans
- Split peas (yellow and green)
- Tofu.

Grains

- Amaranth
- Barley
- Buckwheat
- Millet
- Oats
- Quinoa
- Rice
- Rye
- Spelt
- Teff
- Wheat (organic).

Nuts

- Almonds
- Brazil nuts
- Cashews
- Chestnuts
- Hazelnuts
- Pistachios
- Walnuts.

Seeds

- Chia seeds
- Flax seeds
- Hemp seeds
- Poppy seeds
- Pumpkin seeds
- Sesame seeds (black or white)
- Sunflower seeds.

Herbs and spices

- Allspice
- Basil
- Bay leaf
- Black pepper
- Caraway seeds
- Cardamom
- Cinnamon
- Cloves
- Coriander
- Cumin
- Curry
- Dill
- Fennel
- Fenugreek
- Ginger
- Marjoram
- Mustard seeds
- Nutmeg
- Oregano
- Paprika
- Parsley leaf
- Sage
- Savory
- Star anise
- Thyme
- Turmeric
- Vanilla.

Meat

- Beef
- Bison
- Chicken
- Chicken eggs
- Goat
- Lamb
- Pork
- Turkey
- Venison.

Seafood

Locally harvested, fresh, and sustainable is recommended and will vary depending on geographical location.

- Anchovies
- Crab
- Herring
- Lobster
- Mussels
- Prawns
- Salmon
- Sardines
- Scallops
- Snapper
- Sole
- Trout
- Tuna
- Whitefish.

Breakfast ideas

Warm, nourishing breakfasts are beneficial year-round, but are a necessity in the colder winter months. Hearty nuts, to keep the body warm and strong, as well as seeds are indicated at this time of year.

- Bircher Müesli (see page 171)
- Buttermilk Pancakes (see page 172)
- Millet Muesli (see page 173)
- Nut-Ella, spread on toast (see page 174)
- Scrambled Tofu (see page 175)
- Simple Granola (see page 176).

School lunch and snack ideas

- Apple Muffins (see page 178)
- Applesauce, with a pinch of cinnamon
- Black Bean Brownies (see page 178)
- Bliss Seed Balls (see page 179)
- Candied Ginger (see page 148)
- Chicken-fried rice with a type of bean and quick sautéed spring vegetables that the child enjoys
- Crackers (Homemade), topped with cheese or jam (see page 180)

- Dried fruit
- Hummus (see page 181)
- Kale Sunflower Chips (see page 182)
- Oat and Cardamom Muffins (see page 183)
- Oatmeal and Sesame Chocolate Chip Cookies (see page 184)
- Organic macaroni and cheese
- Pear Juice (see page 185)
- Pear Smoothy (see page 186)
- Peas (Side Dish) (see page 202)
- Popcorn (Homemade), sprinkled with nutritional yeast or cinnamon (see page 186)
- Puffed Amaranth and Seed Bar (see page 187)
- Puffed Lotus Seed with Pumpkin Pie Spice (see page 122)
- Roasted Chickpeas (see page 188)
- Sliced apples, rubbed with a little lemon juice
- Smoked salmon
- Sweet Potato Toast (see page 189)
- Tuna sandwich
- Veggies—all veggies should be cooked
- Whole grain or gluten-free wrap with beans, cheese, cooked seasonal veggies, rice, and yoghurt sauce to spread
- Winter Squash Loaf (see page 191).

Home lunch and dinner ideas

- Anellini Pasta with Broccoli and Ham (see page 192)
- Cabbage, the German Way (see page 193)
- Celeriac (Celery Root) Salad (see page 195)
- Crock Pot Beef and Bean, or only Bean Chili (see page 195)
- Honey and Ginger Wild Salmon (see page 196)
- Leek and Potato Soup (see page 197)
- Lentil Dal (see page 198)
- Millet (Side Dish) (see page 199)
- Millet Soupy Porridge (see page 200)
- Orange Chicken (or Tofu) and Almonds (see page 201)
- Peas (Side Dish) (see page 202)
- Steamed Egg Soup (see page 204)
- Sweet Potato and Butter Bean (Lima Bean) Soup (see page 205)
- Vegetarian Lasagna (see page 206).

CHAPTER 9

Common Childhood Ailments

The five grains are used to nourish, the five fruits to assist, the five animals to fortify, the five vegetables to fulfill. Combining the energetic properties of these in one's diet can reinforce the essence and qi. These five types of food have specific effects and properties. When combined with the principles of the seasons, the five elements, and the pathophysiology of the five Zang organs, one can utilize the methods of dietetics as an adjunct tool to nourish, convalesce, and treat.

Maoshing Ni (1995, p.94)

When diet is wrong, medicine is of no use. When diet is correct, medicine is of no need.

Ayuverdic proverb, quoted in Cantrell (2012)

The goal of following a TCM diet for children is to ultimately reduce the frequency of some of the most common childhood complaints. Nourishing the Spleen, as discussed in Chapter 2, is the root treatment for all the syndromes discussed in this chapter. Since many childhood illnesses stem from a weak and immature digestion, protecting and strengthening it will prevent some of these common ailments from occurring and reduce the frequency and severity of others. Growing up on a dairy farm, I drank a lot of cow's milk. I now know that too much dairy, especially for children, causes phlegm accumulation and is difficult to digest. This caused chronic ear infections and stomach aches, and I remember feeling full and bloated on a regular basis. Most likely, the internal pathway linking the Stomach and Intestines to the inner ears was affected causing the earache. The doctors would prescribe antibiotics for the earache, which would only further weaken my Spleen *Qi*, reinforcing the condition, and it would re-occur. In my case, if I had eliminated dairy for a period of time and added in foods to nourish my Spleen *Qi*, this would have helped to naturally strengthen my digestion, reduced the bloating, and my earache would not have returned. My daughter, who is now seven years old, does not know what an earache is; I attribute this to her diet and her low dairy consumption.

Babies, toddlers, and children are prone to accumulation disorder. Another name for this is food stagnation. This happens when food stops digesting properly and there is a backup through the digestive tract. The Spleen is responsible for transforming and then transporting the food, and if it is not transforming properly (breaking food down), it will also not be able to transport it either, causing food stagnation. This is very commonly seen in children in many of the disorders in this chapter. It can be the root problem in conditions such as constipation, diarrhea, colic, ear infections, asthma, stomach aches, and skin conditions. It is said in TCM that accumulation disorder is the "cause of one hundred diseases."

When choosing the recommendations below for dietary therapy, keep in mind the seasonality of the fruit or vegetable listed and cooking methods suitable for the season. For instance, in the winter, less cold and cooling foods would be indicated, and only a small amount of raw fruit.

Children go through so many different phases of growth spurts and emotional transformations that it is impossible for them to get to adulthood without any illness. Dietary therapy using food commonly found in the kitchen and herbs from a home spice cabinet can, in certain instances, be enough to heal a condition or otherwise offer a form of symptom relief until the body recovers. Optimal health cannot be achieved without dietary adjustment, and when prescribed alongside a TCM treatment will yield improved outcomes. Dietary therapy is one of the eight branches of TCM (along with meditation, exercise, acupuncture, herbal medicine, cosmology, Feng Shui, and massage), and the one branch that must not be left out in the treatment of children.

If using this book without the care of a qualified TCM practitioner, I recommend getting an initial assessment from a family doctor or specialist to rule out a more serious condition.

Health signs that show up on the face

Our faces can reveal a lot about the state or an imbalance in our internal health. Children move so quickly between a state of health, illness, and back

112

again that many of these signs do not have a chance to manifest as they would on an adult who has longstanding health issues. However, there are a few things, that when they do show up, should be paid attention to:

- **Blue vein at the bridge of the nose:** This will usually show up in babies or children under the age of six, although I have seen it in slightly older children. This can manifest for a few different reasons, but since this area of the face relates to the Spleen or pancreas, it has to do with processing food, usually sugars. A baby could have this vein if the mother had gestational diabetes or a high sugar intake during pregnancy. A child could have this vein if their sugar intake is too high, or they are not metabolizing it well. A child could also have a food allergy to wheat, eggs, soy, or any other common allergen.
- **Area above the mouth:** The area above the lips shows the state of the Stomach function. A nice plump area here shows good Stomach *Qi*. If it is sunken, this would show the need to nourish the Stomach *Qi*, and the child may have issues with their digestive health, such as low appetite, stomach pain, or bloating.
- **Lips:** A refined upper lip area, with sharper tips along the lip line, shows a child with a very refined palate. They will taste food strongly and may tend to be picky eaters. A child with a rounded and smoother upper lip line will not have this strong palate and may eat a wider variety of foods.
- **Ear tips:** The tip of children's ears may get red if they eat a food they have an allergy or sensitivity to.

Dosages for herbal teas

When utilizing herbal teas for an acute condition, treatment can be discontinued as soon as the child is feeling better. Herbal teas are milder than TCM formulas, with dosing dependent on the condition, and I have listed this information below. In general, dosing for children for herbal teas is as follows:

Age	Dosage
Younger than 2 years	½ to 1 teaspoon
2–4 years	2 teaspoons
4–7 years	1 tablespoon
7–11 years	2 tablespoons

Constipation

Constipation is one of the more commonly seen issues in children. In TCM, having a daily bowel movement is considered normal. Anything less than that can be considered constipation; Western medicine, on the other hand, only classifies constipation if there are less than four bowel movements a week. Babies and toddlers usually have more frequent movements, ranging anywhere between one to five times daily. It is important with constipation to assess any deviation from the norm in the child and to be striving for at least once-a-day elimination. Along with normal appetite, and an absence from any discomfort along the gastrointestinal (GI) tract, optimal bowel movements are a sign of a healthy functioning digestive system.

A child who has experienced constipation may start to withhold their feces due to fear of the pain that a previous movement has caused. They may fear public washrooms or not want to take the time when they feel the urge because life is too fun to stop playing to go to the washroom. Withholding then becomes a vicious cycle; it causes a buildup of stools in the lower bowel, causing fecal impaction and potentially encopresis (when a runny stool escapes through the impacted feces, soiling the underwear). This necessitates diagnosis from a specialist, but dietary changes are still required as the root treatment. In this case, it is also worth looking at any life changes that may have occurred in the recent past. The Large Intestine is responsible for "letting go" of the waste that does not serve us anymore. Maybe the child is having trouble "letting go" of Mom and Dad while attending daycare, or "letting go" of their pacifier that they found so soothing. It is helpful to investigate this avenue as the emotional component may require input or help from a child expert.

For dietary purposes, I break down constipation into either the excess or deficient type. Excess-type constipation for babies and infants can occur due to accumulation disorder; in older children, accumulation disorder shows up as Heat and Stagnation in the Intestines. Deficiency-type constipation can occur due to Spleen deficiency, where there is not enough Qi to move the bowels through the Intestines; older children may also be deficient in Blood whereby the Blood does not moisten the Intestines, causing dryness.

Excess-type constipation

- Constipation that lasts a few days.
- Foul-smelling breath.

- Distended abdomen.
- Irritable.
- Red cheeks.

With this type of constipation, the parents or caregivers should make sure that the child is not overeating. Overeating creates accumulation disorder and causes heat to build up in the digestive tract. Mindlessly eating while watching television, playing video games, or over-snacking in between meals are some ways children can overeat. "Snacking" has become mainstream nowadays, with any food imaginable wrapped up in a convenient, brightly colored, mini-sized, version of itself, ready to eat. These are irresistible to kids! Reduce the amount of processed "dry" snacks in their diet—crackers, chips, and pretzels.

It is commonly thought to be advantageous to give children raw vegetables when they are constipated due to the fiber content, but because raw vegetables are hard for children to digest, they should be avoided in this case. Most of their vegetables should be cooked, but as the bowels become regular, a small of amount of raw vegetables may be incorporated back into their diet. Cow's milk and milk products can be eliminated for a two-week trial, as certain children are unable to digest the proteins in the milk.

DIETARY THERAPY

- ✓ **Increase fiber:** opt for whole grain versions of bread, pasta, and dough, use whole grains in cooking such as millet, barley, and oats, and make sure most **vegetables are cooked. Pulses** are high in fiber: all beans, peas, and lentils. **Homemade popcorn**, loved by most children, is also remarkably high in fiber.
- ✓ **Avocados** have a cooling thermal nature, are high in fiber, and lubricate the intestines.
- ✓ **Chia seeds** are high in fiber, have a downward-moving action, and are the richest plant source of Omega-3 fatty acids. They lubricate dryness in the body and have a neutral thermal nature. See below for a recipe using chia seeds.

CHIA PUDDING
Ingredients
- ¼ cup of chia seeds
- 1 cup of water or milk of your choice

Method
1. Soak the chia seeds in the water or milk.
2. Let sit for 20 minutes until a gel-like consistency develops.
3. This chia water mixture can be stored refrigerated for up to five days, and can then be eaten with fruit or stirred into soups or eaten as it is, with a little sweetener. Make sure it is room temperature before consuming.

✓ **Flax seeds** have a neutral thermal nature. They are also high in Omega-3 fatty acids and are a known natural laxative. They are best ground just before eating, to ensure they are digested.

✓ **Hemp seeds** have been traditionally used in TCM to relieve constipation. They are sweet in flavor and have a neutral thermal nature.

✓ **Honey** moistens the Large Intestine and has a neutral thermal nature. Local, unpasteurized honey is recommended, as many of the health benefits are lost when heated during pasteurization. Children under one year should not be given honey due to the potential for infant botulism caused by the *Clostridium botulinum* spores in both pasteurized and unpasteurized honey.

✓ **Pears** have a cooling thermal nature, are high in fiber, and are used in TCM for constipation.

✓ **Make sure fluid intake is sufficient.** This will depend on whether it is summer or winter and the child's activity level. Plain, room temperature water throughout the day is recommended. Soups and fruit are hydrating and also helpful.

✓ **Add a few pieces of dried fruit to the diet daily.** Choose dried fruit that is sulfate-free and also free of chemicals. Sulfur dioxide is added to dried fruits to preserve the fruit's original color and to increase its shelf life; naturally dried fruit will be darker in color and can be refrigerated to keep longer. Prunes are a well-known remedy for constipation (see below for the **Prune Puree** recipe); one or two per day should be sufficient. In TCM they are considered cooling and promote the production of Body Fluids. Children under the age of one should only have a small amount, as too many prunes may cause diarrhea due to their cooling nature. Toddlers over the age of one can eat pureed prunes, and older children (age two+) can eat dried fruit.

PRUNE PUREE

Ingredients
- A handful of dried prunes
- Just-boiled water

Method
1. Cover the prunes with boiled water for about 15–30 minutes.
2. Blend the prunes in a food processor to make the puree—both the prunes and the water used to soak them.

✓ **Incorporate fermented foods daily** to help increase beneficial bacteria. Fermented foods include water kefir, tempeh, kombucha, fermented pickles, true sourdough bread, and miso.

+ Watch for overeating.
+ Watch for "dry" food intake such as crackers, chips, and pretzels.

Deficient type constipation

- Can go five to seven days without passing a stool.
- Low appetite.
- May have a sore tummy.
- Fatigue.
- Condition gets worse when tired or with a busy schedule.
- Stools not smelly.
- Blue vein at the bridge of the nose.

This type of constipation is due to Spleen *Qi* deficiency. Lack of energy is present in the body and there is not enough energy to move the food through the digestive tract. Following the Spleen nourishing diet is important to treat the root condition. It is also important to pay attention to eating at regular times of the day and to reduce snacking, which will help prevent overeating, which further burdens the Spleen energy. Eliminating foods that are difficult to digest, such as peanuts, dairy, raw foods, and an excess of sugar and tropical fruits, is indicated.

DIETARY THERAPY

- ✓ **Nourish Spleen *Qi*.**
- ✓ Utilize the properties of the **warming spices** listed below in cooking to stimulate digestion:

  - Aniseed
  - Basil
  - Bay leaf
  - Caraway
  - Cardamom
  - Chives
  - Cinnamon twigs
  - Cumin
  - Ginger
  - Fennel seeds
  - Paprika
  - Parsley
  - Rosemary
  - Savory
  - Tarragon.

- ✓ **Cooked carrots** nourish the Spleen and lubricate the Intestines.
- ✓ **Honey** nourishes the Spleen and Stomach and has a neutral thermal energy. It lubricates the Large Intestine to help with constipation.
- ✓ **Sesame oil** added to cooking promotes bowel movements. It is cool in nature.
- ✓ **Seeds** are lubricating and help to move the stool. If there are undigested seeds in the child's stool, this means they are not digesting them properly; pre-soaking seeds will help with this.
- ✓ **Incorporate more downtime** for the child for unstructured play and rest.

Loose stools

For the purposes of dietary therapy, I will be discussing chronic loose stools here as opposed to acute diarrhea. Acute diarrhea due to a viral or bacterial infection will usually clear up in a few days—diarrhea is the body's way of eliminating the virus or bacteria as quickly as possible. If a baby is six months or younger, always refer the parent to a medical doctor. In babies and children older than six months, a referral to a medical doctor is necessary when the diarrhea is accompanied by a high fever, frequent vomiting, severe pain in the abdomen or rectum, stools with blood or pus, stools that are black and tarry, or symptoms of dehydration. To help the child's body recover from acute diarrhea and to prevent dehydration, **Rice Water** (see below) has been studied to be more effective than an electrolyte solution in reducing the number of stools and rehydrating the body (El Faki, Babikir, and Ali 2001;

Wong 1981). This remedy works remarkably well and quickly for diarrhea, and may also be used for chronic loose stools.

RICE WATER
Ingredients
- ½ cup of uncooked rice (brown or white)
- 8 cups of water

Method
1. Rinse the rice.
2. Add the rice and water to a saucepan and bring to a boil. Stir to prevent the rice sticking.
3. Boil over a medium heat for about 10 minutes. The rice will not be cooked, and the water should not be too starchy. Add more water if this is the case.
4. Strain the water from the rice. Let the rice water cool before drinking.

There can be occasional loose stools in children due to eating very cold, chilled food or drinks, and ingesting an excess of raw foods. A friend's 14-year-old son experienced this while visiting the Royal Tyrrell Museum in Drumheller, Alberta. A typical summer day is hot and dry, and along the way to the museum my friend bought her son a large ice-cold Slurpee (also known as an ICEE, or a Slush drink) to "keep cool." He drank the whole thing quickly, then, while touring the museum, started to feel cramping pain in his lower abdomen. The diarrhea came on so suddenly, he did not have time to make it to a toilet, and, well, you can figure out the embarrassing scenario that unfolded. We found out afterwards that this a common occurrence at the museum and they keep spare shorts on hand for this reason! The combination of extremely hot days with gas stations (petrol stations) en route to the museum serving chilled beverages is a recipe for cold invading the Stomach and Intestines. To recover from this kind of diarrhea, avoid cold, chilled, and raw foods in the diet for a few days, and include warm, cooked foods only.

Food intolerances can also cause loose stools. An intolerance is the inability to digest or absorb certain foods. Intolerance to lactose is common as the lactase enzyme can start to decrease after the age of two. In *Keeping Your Child Healthy with Chinese Medicine*, Bob Flaws states,

According to Western medicine, persistent diarrhea in infants may be due to an adverse reaction to wheat gluten, insufficiency in pancreatic enzymes, sugar malabsorption, and food allergies. Pancreatic enzymes are very much related to the Chinese idea of Spleen function, some Western authors saying the Chinese medical concept of the Spleen should be called the Spleen-pancreas. The clear, bland diet of Chinese Medicine for babies is mostly a wheat-free diet. Sugar malabsorption and food allergies are also addressed by the clear, bland diet and Chinese Herbal medicine. (Flaws 1996, p.80)

All the symptoms of food intolerance (bloating, stomach pain, and loose stools) are indicative of Spleen *Qi* deficiency and should lessen with TCM treatment and dietary adjustments.

For the purposes of dietary therapy, I will cover excess-type and deficient-type loose stools here, which are quite similar in etiology to constipation.

Excess-type loose stools

- Bad breath.
- Foul-smelling stools with undigested food.
- Stools five to six times per day or more.
- Nausea.
- Abdominal bloating.

Excess-type loose stools have their roots in overeating, as does excess-type constipation. Snacking too much between meals or mindlessly eating while watching television or playing video games needs to be addressed. This type of accumulation disorder can also arise from breastfeeding on demand and the baby not being able to fully digest the excess amounts. Breast-fed babies on average have more stools per day than formula-fed babies, and it is important to monitor what is normal for the baby and to look for increases in movements outside of individual norms. As babies grow, the number of stools they have daily starts to reduce, especially when they start on solid foods.

In older children, Liver *Qi* stagnation attacking the Spleen can be a cause of loose stools. Sometimes the loose stools will alternate with constipation. There might be some cramping pain before the movement, and this would occur more frequently when the child is emotionally stressed or upset. In this case, it is still important to nourish Spleen *Qi* as a root condition, and to make sure that greasy (French fries, pizza, potato chips) and excess fatty foods are reduced (too many nuts, too much processed meat). Find out how often over-the-counter drugs and medications (acetaminophen, ibuprofen) are given, as an excess of these can be a contributing factor.

DIETARY THERAPY

✓ Eat at **regular times** each day.
✓ Over time, excess type loose stools can lead to Spleen *Qi* deficiency. Always **nourish Spleen *Qi*** in children to strengthen the root condition. **Rule out food intolerances.** The best way is to keep a food journal for the child to identify a pattern. Symptoms usually begin closer to when the food was ingested, but can also take up to two days to appear.
✓ **Apples** strengthen the Intestines and are a remedy for diarrhea.
✓ **Black pepper** is warming, and added to cooking will help with watery stools.

+ Large amounts of water or fruit juice can be a problem; fruit juice is not recommended for children in TCM due to its cold thermal nature and high sugar content.
+ Overeating—limit snacking.
+ Reduce greasy, fatty foods.

Deficient-type loose stools

* Fatigue.
* Chronic loose stools.
* Low appetite.
* Loose, watery stools.
* Cramping pains in abdomen.
* Stools have little to no smell.
* Loose stools after a meal.
* Blue vein at the bridge of the nose.

Deficient-type loose stools come from a Spleen *Qi* deficiency. The Spleen is too weak to digest foods and drinks properly and they are not separated properly from pure and impure; the stools are then unformed and released easily and often. This will take a little more time to resolve, and any foods that have downward-moving action and that are lubricating should be avoided until the digestion strengthens.

- ✓ Follow a **Spleen _Qi_ nourishing diet.**
- ✓ **Apples** strengthen the Intestines and are a remedy for diarrhea.
- ✓ **Barley** strengthens the Spleen and treats diarrhea if it is pan-roasted first before cooking.
- ✓ **Dried licorice:** children can suck on the dried root, or it can be brewed into tea.
- ✓ **Lotus seeds** (found in the Asian food aisle at the grocery store) strengthen the Spleen and astringe chronic loose stools. See below for a recipe using lotus seeds.
- ✓ **Add a pinch of nutmeg** to food (oatmeal, muffins, pancakes, toast). Nutmeg astringes the Large Intestine and warms the Spleen and Stomach.
- ✓ **Rice congee** is one of the easiest meals to digest and nourishes the Middle Burner (Spleen and Stomach) (see the recipe for **Ginger and Rice Congee below**).

Avoid or eliminate:

- + Raw, cold food and cold drinks.
- + Reduce or eliminate honey as it is a strong lubricant for the intestines.
- + Reduce or eliminate spinach as it is a strong lubricant for the intestines.

PUFFED LOTUS SEEDS WITH PUMPKIN PIE SPICE

Similar in taste to popcorn, puffed lotus seeds are easy to make, store well, can be eaten as a snack, and are beneficial for children with chronic loose stools. Lotus seeds are neutral, sweet and not only nourish the Spleen, but also the Kidneys, and the Heart and calms the spirit. Can also be found in Indian speciality food stores as _makhana_.

Ingredients
- 3 cups of puffed lotus seeds
- 2–3 tbsp ghee, oil, or butter
- 2 tsp pumpkin spice blend (1 tsp cinnamon, ½ tsp nutmeg, ¼ tsp ground ginger, ⅛ tsp ground cloves, all blended together)

Method
1. Heat a heavy-bottomed saucepan.

2. Add the ghee or butter and puffed lotus seeds and roast them over a low heat for about 8–9 minutes, stirring continuously until they have a nice crunch.
3. Stir through the pumpkin pie spice blend and stir for one minute.
4. Turn off the heat.
5. Transfer to a container or bowl and let cool.

Common cold and influenza

Common colds are just that. Common. Most children will get at least one cold per season, and if a child is starting daycare, there will be more exposure and greater chances of acquiring the virus. Influenza viruses are more prevalent in the fall and winter and in children may include diarrhea and vomiting. Prevention of the common cold and influenza by strengthening the Defensive Qi (Wei Qi) and immune system is the first thing we would want to address if the child catches colds or flus frequently and/or does not recover in a normal amount of time. Symptoms of a cold usually peak within a few days but can last anywhere from 10 to 14 days. The common cold or common acute upper respiratory tract infection is an acute viral infectious disease of the upper respiratory tract. Symptoms can include a sore throat, stuffy or runny nose, cough, and malaise. There is no "cure" or any effective antiviral that can be given by orthodox medicine for the common cold, and, as such, treatment is focused on symptom relief. Influenza will hit very quickly and symptoms of a fever, headache, muscle pain, cough, and sore throat last for about 4 to 8 days, with symptoms decreasing after that. Weakness, fatigue, and a cough could last several weeks post-influenza. Tamiflu is an antiviral that works by attacking the flu virus to prevent it from multiplying in the body if taken within 48 hours at the onset of symptoms. One of the principle active ingredients in Tamiflu is shikimic acid, which is derived from star anise.

In TCM the common cold and influenza are external pathogenic factors, and the more commonly seen are wind-cold and wind-heat. As with any external pathogenic factor, the focus for herbs and dietary therapy is to use pungent and dispersing foods to push the pathogenic factors out of the body. Over-the-counter cold and cough medications should never be given to children under the age of six. In 2009 Health Canada conducted a review and found that these products have not been shown to be effective but can instead cause serious harm, including overdose and side effects.[1]

Children will be more prone to acquiring a wind-cold or wind-heat

---

1 See www.healthycanadians.gc.ca/recall-alert-rappel-avis/hc-sc/2016/57622a-eng.php

condition due to their immature internal organs and especially if they have had poor diet, lack of sleep, or long exposure to cold and/or windy weather without proper clothing protection.

When a cough accompanies an external pathogenic factor, it is considered an acute cough. It can turn into a chronic cough if the pathogenic factor is not fully resolved and the child's cough comes and goes. This is discussed under "Chronic coughs" below. Coughs can be a source of anxiety for parents, and are a major reason for Emergency Room visits. It is difficult to listen to your young child waking through the night with fits of coughing, and it can become tiring when it happens over several nights to weeks. There are a few effective diet remedies that can be given at home to help soothe the respiratory tract and reduce phlegm if needed.

Wind-cold

- Aversion to cold.
- Chills.
- Low or no fever.
- No sweat.
- Headache.
- Body aches.
- A cough.
- Sneezing.
- Runny nose with slight clear or white discharge.

WIND-COLD COUGH

- A cough with thin, white, or clear mucus.

Honey before bed for a nocturnal cough has been researched to be more effective than no treatment. It was also shown to be more effective than dextromethorphan for symptomatic relief with no side effects (Paul *et al.* 2007). A second, well-designed, randomized control trial also found honey to be effective for upper respiratory infections—1½ tsp was given 30 minutes before bedtime for the study (Ashkin and Mounsey 2013). I would suggest using raw honey, as it has not been pasteurized and has a stronger antibacterial effect. For wind-cold coughs in children over the age of one, dissolve 1½ tsp of raw honey into a little cup of warm water for them to drink before bed.

Unpasteurized honey has antibacterial, anti-inflammatory, and immune-boosting properties.

DIETARY THERAPY

Dietary therapy for wind-cold involves using warm and pungent food and herbs: ginger, scallions (also known as green onions or spring onions), cinnamon, garlic, and pepper have all been traditionally used (see the recipes for **Ginger or Scallion Tea** and **Cinnamon Oatmeal** below). Rosemary resolves the exterior and can also be used for common cold.

GINGER OR SCALLION TEA

This is the most traditional TCM remedy to take at the onset of a wind-cold attack and regularly until a sweat has been induced and symptoms start to ease. See above for dosage instructions. The ingredients can be found at every grocery store. The added sweetener should make it palatable for children.

Ingredients
- 4 pieces of fresh ginger, sliced, with skin on (about ¼ inch thick)
- 2 tbsp scallions, chopped (white/light green part only)
- 1 tbsp raw sugar or honey
- 4 cups of water

Method
1. Bring the water to a boil in a saucepan.
2. Place the sliced ginger and scallions in the water. Turn the heat to low and simmer for about 10–15 minutes.
3. Strain the ginger and scallions, reserving the water (tea).
4. Add raw sugar or honey to the tea, and serve a few times daily, until the cold or flu symptoms ease.
5. Reheat the tea as needed.
6. You could also wrap the child in blankets and allow them to sweat.

Garlic, cinnamon, and ginger all have antiviral and antibiotic effects.

CINNAMON OATMEAL

Oats are warming and easy to digest when sick. Cinnamon and ginger are both warm and pungent and help to release the pathogen.

Ingredients
- ½ cup of rolled oats
- 1½ cups of water
- 1 tsp cinnamon
- ½ tsp dried ginger
- Honey to sweeten

Method
1. Add the oats to water in a saucepan. Bring to a boil over a medium to high heat.
2. Boil and stir regularly for 5 minutes.
3. Remove from the heat and stir in the cinnamon, ginger, and honey, to taste.

Avoid or eliminate:

+ Cold foods (dairy, tropical fruit, food straight out of the fridge, raw vegetables).
+ Greasy, difficult to digest foods.

Wind-heat

- Fever and chills (more fever than chills).
- Slight sweating.
- Runny nose with yellow discharge.
- A cough.
- Sore throat.
- Thirst.

WIND-HEAT COUGH

- A cough with yellow, sticky phlegm.

Use 1½ tsp of honey as indicated for a wind-cold cough, but with a wind-heat cough you would also want to try and clear the heat. Dissolve the honey in a little bit of warm mint tea and give to the child before bed. Marjoram, spearmint, peppermint, lemongrass, or a dosage of **Elderberry Syrup** (see below) (which contains honey) can also be used as they are all cooling.

DIETARY THERAPY

Use cooling and pungent food and herbs. Children are more prone to wind-heat than wind-cold due to their naturally *Yang* constitutions. Influenza will manifest primarily as wind-heat. Serve tea regularly until a fever breaks and symptoms start to ease. See above for dosage instructions.

Mint is cooling, aromatic and pungent. It disperses wind-heat, cools the head, and benefits the throat. Marjoram, spearmint, peppermint, and lemongrass may also be used in its place, as they are all cooling and pungent.

MINT TEA

Ingredients
- 15–20 fresh mint leaves (or 1½ tbsp dried mint)
- 2 cups of water
- Honey to sweeten, if needed
- (You can also use a mint teabag if no fresh or dried mint is available)

Method
1. Bring the water to a boil in a small saucepan.
2. Remove from the heat, stir in the mint, cover with a lid and allow to steep, for 10–15 minutes.
3. Strain the mint leaves and add honey if required.
4. Have the child drink regularly at the onset of symptoms.

ELDERBERRY SYRUP

This recipe makes about three cups of syrup. Store refrigerated. The syrup lasts for about six months, but check for mold before serving. For store-bought versions, check recommendations on the label.

Dosage

- Up to 4 years of age: 1 tsp per day.
- Age 5–9: 1 tsp, 2 x daily.
- Age 10–14: 1 tsp, 2–4 x daily.

These wonderful berries are easy to find, they are antiviral, and the best thing about them for children is that they taste delicious! Elderberries have been studied to effectively shorten the duration of illness and to also treat upper respiratory infections (Hawkins *et al.* 2019; Torabian *et al.* 2019). They have heat clearing properties, nourish the lungs, and resolve wind and phlegm. Here is a recipe for making elderberry syrup if you can harvest your own, otherwise the syrups are now widely available in health food sections and stores.

Ingredients

- 2 cups of dried elderberries (or 4 cups of fresh berries)
- 4 cups of water
- 1 cup of raw honey (or use maple syrup if vegan or for children under the age of one year)

Method

1. Add the elderberries to the water in a saucepan.
2. Bring the water to a boil. Reduce the heat and allow to simmer for about 30–40 minutes.
3. Do not cover the pan and make sure to simmer for the full length of time, to eliminate the cyanide-like toxin in the seeds.
4. Remove from the heat and steep for one hour.
5. Once cooled, strain through a cheesecloth, then add the honey or maple syrup, and stir to combine.
6. Store in a sterilized glass jar in the refrigerator.

Chronic cough

It is not commonly recognized in our Western society that most coughs in children are diet-induced and/or do not improve due to the diet. Acute coughs that turn into chronic coughs are a common pediatric complaint, and parents are usually quick to reassure others that their child is not contagious, "Don't worry, my child isn't sick; he/she has had this cough for weeks." The Spleen, the root of digestion, when impaired, causes phlegm production. There is a saying in TCM, "the Earth element (Spleen) creates damp and the Metal element (Lungs) stores it." The Lungs are delicate organs to begin with and especially so in children due to being immature. If children develop an external pathogenic factor, they are likely to develop a cough along with it. These coughs will usually eventually resolve on their own with proper rest, diet, and time. Chronic coughs, on the other hand, are due to an internal pattern and will usually require some treatment and dietary shift to resolve. There is a close connection between the Lungs and Spleen, so when the Lungs are compromised due to a cough, the Spleen, which is already inherently weaker in children to begin with, can become even weaker than normal and allow phlegm accumulation.

Phlegm accumulation in the lungs

- A cough with mucus that can be heard in the lungs.
- Rough breathing.
- Paroxysmal coughing.
- The cough is usually worse at night and first thing in the morning.

DIETARY THERAPY

Dietary therapy for phlegm accumulation is much more effective if certain foods are reduced or eliminated in the diet to help the Spleen regain its strength and to stop it from producing more mucus. Bitter and pungent foods will help to drain and eliminate phlegm.

- ✓ **Spleen Qi nourishing diet.**
- ✓ **Clear, bland diet.**

Neutral thermal nature—can be applied for both phlegm accumulation with and without heat:

- **Turnip:** enters the Lung and resolves phlegm. A few slices of raw turnip are more useful to cut through mucus if a child will eat them as such.

Warming thermal nature—helpful for phlegm with no heat signs:

- **Basil:** pungent and warming; enters the Lungs.
- **Cardamom:** warming and drying, goes to the Lungs and resolves phlegm. Stimulates digestion.
- **Cinnamon:** pungent and warming.
- **Dried citrus peel brewed as tea** (can make at home with unsprayed tangerine or mandarin orange peel): warming, transforms phlegm, and descends Lung *Qi*.
- **Ginger:** enters the Spleen, Stomach, and Lung, and transforms phlegm.

- **Thyme:** transforms phlegm, warms the lung, and suppresses a cough.

Cooling thermal nature—helpful for phlegm with heat signs:

- **Lemon:** cooling, transforms phlegm, and stops a cough.
- **Pears:** clear heat, resolve phlegm, and go to the Lungs.
- **Peppermint:** clears heat, pungent, loosens phlegm.
- **Radishes:** pungent, affect the Lungs and Stomach and transform thick mucus conditions.

Until phlegm has cleared, avoid or eliminate:

+ Cold, chilled food or drink like ice cream, popsicles, or refrigerated beverages.
+ Dairy.
+ Greasy, deep-fried foods.
+ Tropical fruit.
+ Especially damp-forming foods, such as roasted peanut butter, tomato sauce, eggs, or an excess of nuts.
+ Excess sugar.

LUNG AND SPLEEN *QI* DEFICIENCY COUGH

- A cough with thin white phlegm.
- Shortness of breath.
- Easily catches a cold.
- Low appetite.
- Easily fatigued.
- Pale face.
- The cough gets worse with activity.

DIETARY THERAPY

- ✓ **Spleen Qi nourishing diet:** make sure to include aromatic spices and herbs.
- ✓ **Clear, bland diet** until condition improves.
- ✓ **Warm, cooked foods** primarily until condition improves.
- ✓ **Almonds:** benefit the Lungs. Can use almond milk.
- ✓ **Apples:** cooling thermal nature; enter the Lungs and benefit the Lungs.
- ✓ **Apricots (dried or fresh):** neutral thermal nature; enter the Lungs and benefit the Lungs.

✓ **Carrots (cooked):** neutral thermal nature; benefit a cough and nourish the Middle Burner.

✓ **Grapes:** neutral thermal nature; benefit a Lung deficiency cough.

✓ **Job's tears** (also known as Chinese pearl barley or Coix seed) is gluten-free (unlike pearl barley), sweet and bland, strengthens the Spleen and Lungs, and removes excess fluid. See below for a recipe using Job's tears.

✓ **Pears: see the recipe for Pear Smoothy** (page 186).

SIMPLE JOB'S TEARS PORRIDGE

Ingredients
- ½ cup of Job's tears (Chinese pearl barley)
- 6 cups of water
- Raw cane sugar or honey, to taste

Method
1. Rinse the Job's tears and add to a saucepan along with the water.
2. Bring to a boil, then reduce the heat and simmer for about an hour.
3. Add cane sugar or honey to taste, and serve warm.

Avoid or eliminate:

+ Cold, chilled foods like ice cream or popsicles.
+ Dairy.
+ Greasy, deep-fried foods.
+ Tropical fruit.
+ Especially damp-forming foods, such as roasted peanut butter, tomato sauce, eggs, or an excess of nuts.
+ Excess sugar or fruit juice.

Eczema

Eczema (also known as atopic dermatitis) is a common inflammatory skin condition in children. It is characterized by:

• Itch (can be severe and the child will scratch until the skin bleeds).
• Redness.
• Skin that is very dry or scaly.
• Open, crusted, or weeping sores.

We now know that the presence of atopic eczema implicates a greater chance of developing a food allergy—there is evidence that eczema can somehow trigger a food allergy (Tsakok *et al.* 2017). Known as the "atopic march," infants who develop eczema have a higher likelihood of developing food allergies, hay fever, and asthma as they grow older. Because the skin is cracked, food particles are introduced through the skin rather than through the digestive tract, and are much more likely to cause allergies (Leung *et al.* 2019). If you have ever watched an infant eat, you know that more food ends up on their bodies than in their mouths! This "atopic march" makes preventing and treating atopic eczema a top priority in the future health of a child. The initial signs of eczema could show up after the first vaccination due to the heat toxins that are introduced into the system, or when cow's milk is first introduced due to its cold nature and the accumulation of phlegm.

If a child is being breast-fed, the mother's diet should also be assessed and may need to be modified to either rule out or confirm what is a contributing factor to the child's eczema. Eliminating dairy, eggs, wheat, nuts, soy, harmful food additives (MSG, food coloring, flavoring, artificial sweeteners, preservatives), and an excess of deep-fried or spicy foods for at least two weeks will help to identify potential allergens—by two weeks, the proteins will no longer be present in breast milk. Dairy can be reintroduced first to test as a causative factor, as this is the most common allergen.

The Spleen, being immature in children, is easily overwhelmed by a faulty diet, and in the acute phase of eczema the damp-heat smolders under the skin. Symptoms of this phase are:

- Sudden appearance.
- Appearing anywhere on the body.
- A red rash that may be blistered and swollen.
- Open, crusted, or weepy sores.
- Intense itching.

The chronic form of eczema is due to Spleen and Blood deficiency. This form evolves from the acute stage due to the heat eventually drying out the skin or it can also happen due to a child's Spleen *Qi* deficiency and weakness leading to blood deficiency dryness. The blood is responsible for nourishing and hydrating the skin. Symptoms of this phase are:

- A rash that is scaly and hard.
- Mild itching.
- Skin can feel rough and dry.

DIETARY THERAPY

With eczema there is always dampness present in varying degrees and Spleen *Qi* deficiency. Both need to be addressed in the diet alongside treatment of eczema for long-term results. If there is a lot of dampness involved, the child will also have other signs of mucus discharge in the sinuses or phlegm in the chest. Although there is heat involved, the root condition requires warming the Spleen and aiding in the transformation of fluids to reduce dampness.

✓ **Nourish Spleen *Qi* diet.**

- **Sunshine:** it has been said that "sunshine is the best medicine," and in this case it holds true. Babies who had *greater* ultraviolet (UV) light exposure in early infancy had lower incidences of eczema and lower levels of immune factors associated with allergic inflammation by six months of age (Rueter *et al.* 2019). Vitamin D supplementation was also tested and showed no significant difference in the outcome for eczema; sunshine was the key factor.

Foods that aid in the transformation of dampness:

- **Legumes:** all legumes transform dampness. They can be drying in excess and less is required if there are not as many signs of dampness or phlegm. Especially nourishing to the Spleen are chickpeas (garbanzo beans), yellow peas, and fava beans.
- **Pearl barley or whole barley:** whole barley is an un-hulled whole grain and more nutritious than pearled barley due to the bran not being removed. Pearl barley is easier to digest in the same way that white rice is compared to brown rice. Pearl barley is still highly nutritious. Both versions nourish the Spleen and Stomach and resolve dampness.
- **Pumpkin:** neutral thermal nature; nourishes the Spleen and Stomach, tonifies *Qi*, and resolves dampness and phlegm.

Foods that nourish the Blood and heal dry skin:

- **Sesame oil:** nourishes the blood and moistens the skin.
- **Spinach:** nourishes the blood and moistens dryness. Do not use with loose stools.
- **Nettles:** nourish and cleanse the Blood and drain dampness.

External poultice: grate a raw potato, wrap it in a damp paper towel, cheesecloth, or thin towel, and place over or apply directly to the eczema patches. Secure with a bandage. Leave in place for 20 minutes at a time, until the skin begins to heal.

Reduce or eliminate:

+ Cold, chilled, or iced food or drink.
+ Dairy.
+ Deep-fried foods.
+ Fruit and vegetable juices.
+ Ice cream.
+ Oranges, bananas, tomatoes, and avocados.
+ Peanut butter or an excess of oily nuts.
+ Shellfish (shrimp, crab, lobster, etc.), which is known in TCM to exacerbate skin conditions.
+ Sugary yoghurt (coconut and dairy).
+ Wheat (an allergen, and damp-forming), refined flour, and sugar, which are all often found in packaged, processed snacks, including baked goods such as muffins, cookies, bagels, crackers, pretzels, breads, cereals, pasta, and cakes.

Allergic rhinitis (hay fever)

Allergic rhinitis is not a serious condition, albeit it is an uncomfortable one. It occurs when the immune system overreacts to particles in the air that are breathed in and causes inflammation in the nose. Common seasonal causes are due to pollen from trees, grasses, weeds, and mold spores, and occur mainly in the spring, summer, and fall. Perennial causes lasting year-round can come from animal dander, dust mites, mold, or food allergies. The goal of TCM is to bring the body into attunement, to reduce, and in the best case, eliminate, the environmental sensitivity in the child.

Common symptoms include:

• Runny (watery nasal discharge) or stuffy nose.
• Sneezing.
• Red, itchy, and watery eyes.
• Itchy throat, mouth, nose, and ears.
• A cough.

DIETARY THERAPY

✓ **Local unpasteurized honey:** micro doses of pollen act as a homeopathic remedy. Children require about 1–2 tbsp per day for a therapeutic effect, which should be started one month before the start of allergy season. One study by Asha'ari *et al.* (2013) found this to be helpful for overall and individual symptoms of allergic rhinitis.

✓ **Omega-3 fatty acids in fish (wild salmon, sardines, mackerel, herring):** may protect against allergic disease. It has been studied to reduce the occurrence of allergic rhinitis in infants. Higher levels of Omega-3 fatty acid in the blood of children aged eight was shown to have a lower incidence of allergic rhinitis by age 16 (D'Vaz *et al.* 2012; Magnusson *et al.* 2017).

✓ **Perilla seed oil:** pungent and warming. Used mainly in Korean cooking. Can be used in vegetarian cooking as a replacement for fish Omega-3. Should not be heated to a high temperature; it is better used non-heated. As shown in studies, it has a high Omega-3 content and may decrease allergic rhinitis, suppressing the production of chemical mediators in allergy responses (Osakabe *et al.* 2004).

Liver heat flaring up

This occurs in the spring when aggravated by exposure to pollen. Clearing Liver heat and calming excess *Yang* is indicated.

DIETARY THERAPY

✓ **Celery:** bitter and cooling; balances the Liver.
✓ **Chrysanthemum tea:** clears the Liver and the eyes, subdues Liver *Yang*. Many tea companies now carry dried chrysanthemum.
✓ **Mint:** clears heat from the head and eyes.
✓ **Nettles:** a natural antihistamine, nettles appear in the early spring, just when they are needed. They clear heat, astringe fluids, and nourish Liver *Yin* to anchor *Yang*.

Avoid or eliminate:

+ Dairy.
+ Deep-fried, greasy foods.

Lung and Spleen Qi deficiency

- Allergy symptoms as above, with acute flare-up, or year-round.
- Easily fatigued.
- Low appetite.
- Pale face.

DIETARY THERAPY

- ✓ **Spleen *Qi* nourishing diet.**
- ✓ **Almonds:** benefit the Lungs. Can use almond milk.
- ✓ **Apples:** cooling thermal nature; enter the Lungs and benefit the Lungs.
- ✓ **Apricots (dried or fresh):** neutral thermal nature; enter the Lungs and benefit the Lungs.

Chronic asthma

Asthma is the most common chronic disease in children, affecting 12.5 percent. Pediatric asthma causes the lungs and airways to become easily inflamed when exposed to certain triggers (pollen, respiratory infection, trigger foods, pollution, animals).

Common symptoms of asthma include:

- Wheezing.
- Shortness of breath.
- A cough.
- Tight feeling in the chest.

It can be incredibly stressful for the parents of a child with asthma as they are uncertain when or what will trigger an asthma attack. Interestingly, asthma rates have been decreasing in some parts of Europe and North America due to the careful and more reserved use of antibiotics in infants. Researchers found that a reduction in antibiotic prescriptions for infants under the age of one year resulted in a reduced incidence of asthma by age five (Patrick *et al.* 2020). Since a low microbiome has been linked to asthma, not disrupting the sensitive system at a young age seems to be a preventative measure (Abrahamsson *et al.* 2014). Another study conducted with 598 Dutch school-age children, ages 8–13, found that a diet high in whole grain products and fish seems to have a reduced risk of developing asthma. Whole grains and fish were linked to a reduction of 54 percent and 66 percent respectively for asthma and 45 percent and 56 percent for wheezing. This study did not find fish oil supplements to be of any benefit (Tabak *et al.* 2006).

Fish oil supplementation was also not shown to be a protective factor in the development of asthma in a study in 2019 from Sweden (Klingberg, Brekke, and Ludvigsson 2019); again, it was eating actual fish that offered benefit. This study found that the early and intermediate introduction of fish into the diet as compared to late introduction was consistently associated with a decreased risk of asthma. The study also found that the early introduction of infant formula in combination with a short breastfeeding time *increases* the risk of asthma (Klingberg *et al.* 2019). This was also found to be true when Australian children who had early introduction of MOTBM (milk other than breast milk) during the first six months of life had almost double the risk of development of asthma (El-Heneidy *et al.* 2018). We know in TCM that cow milk and soy, the main ingredient in most infant formulas, generates damp and phlegm in the body that goes into the lungs, so these studies are consistent with TCM theory.

Diet is an important factor in the treatment and prevention of asthma, and parents and children alike will be motivated to continue these eating patterns once they see reduced symptoms and less frequent attacks. There are several different etiologies for pediatric asthma in TCM. There is always a Lung deficiency, along with also Spleen and/or Kidney deficiency. Liver *Qi* can stagnate and affect the Lungs. The underlying condition for each etiology is one of Lung deficiency requiring nourishment. There is also excess due to the phlegm that is involved, derived from a deficient Spleen *Qi*. Foods that nourish the Lungs are indicated, phlegm and damp-producing food greatly reduced or eliminated, phlegm and damp-reducing foods included, and the Spleen and/or Kidneys nourished by diet.

DIETARY THERAPY

- ✓ **Maintain a diverse gut microbiome** (see Chapter 4).
- ✓ **Almonds:** benefit the Lungs. Can use almond milk.
- ✓ **Apples:** cool heat and benefit the Lungs. Research has found benefit in an apple a day to keep asthma away (Boyer and Liu 2004).
- ✓ **Apricots (dried or fresh):** neutral thermal nature; enter the Lungs and benefit the Lungs.
- ✓ **Cardamom:** warming, pungent, stimulates digestion. Exhibits bronchial-dilating effects (Khan, Jabeen, and Gilani 2011).

- ✓ **Dried citrus peel brewed as tea** (can make at home with unsprayed tangerine or mandarin orange peel): warming, transforms phlegm, and descends Lung *Qi*.
- ✓ **Fish:** supplement *Qi* and Blood and studied benefits for asthma.
- ✓ **Ginger (fresh):** benefits the Lungs, transforms phlegm.
- ✓ **Pears:** benefit the Lungs, clear heat, transform phlegm.
- ✓ **Perilla seed oil:** pungent and warming. Used mainly in Korean cooking. Can be used in vegetarian cooking as a replacement for fish Omega-3. Should not be heated to a high temperature; it is better used non-heated. It has a high Omega-3 content and has been shown to have a positive effect on allergic inflammation in asthmatic mice (Chang, Chen, and Lin 2012).
- ✓ **Turnips:** enter the Lung and resolve phlegm. A few slices of raw turnip are more useful to cut through mucus if a child will eat them as such.
- ✓ **Whole grains** (supplement Spleen Earth): amaranth, barley, buckwheat, millet, oats, rye, spelt, quinoa.

Avoid:

- + Infant formula for the first six months of life. According to TCM theory, goat formulas are less phlegm-forming.
- + Antibiotics under the age of one year.

Reduce or eliminate:

- + Chilled, iced, or frozen food and drink.
- + Dairy.
- + Deep-fried foods.
- + Fruit juices.
- + Ice cream.
- + Oranges, bananas, tomatoes, avocados.
- + Peanut butter or an excess of oily nuts.
- + Sugary yoghurts (coconut and dairy).
- + Wheat (allergen, and damp-forming), refined flour, and sugar, which are all often found in packaged, processed snacks, including baked goods such as muffins, cookies, bagels, crackers, pretzels, breads, cereals, pasta, and cakes.

Lung deficiency

- Frequently catches colds.
- Short of breath.
- Worse with exercise or exposure to cold air.

DIETARY THERAPY

✓ All the above **dietary recommendations for asthma** should be followed.

Lung and Spleen Qi deficiency

- Asthma symptoms.
- Low appetite.
- Fatigue.
- Frequent colds.
- Chronic productive cough.
- Copious clear phlegm.

DIETARY THERAPY

✓ All the above **dietary recommendations for asthma** should be followed, along with a **nourishing Spleen *Qi*** diet.

Lung and Kidney deficiency

- Asthma symptoms.
- Dark circles under the eyes.
- Cold feet or lower back.
- Congenital weakness or illness.

DIETARY THERAPY

✓ All the above **dietary recommendations for asthma** should be followed, along with **nourishing the Kidneys.**
✓ **All black foods nourish the Kidneys:** black soybeans, black beans, blackberries, seaweed, blueberries.
✓ **Black sesame seeds:** strengthen the Kidneys.

✓ **Bone broths:** the minerals in bone broths deeply nourish the Kidneys.

✓ **Chestnuts:** strengthen both the Spleen and the Kidneys.

✓ **Lentils:** increase the *Jing* (Essence) of the Kidneys.

✓ **Millet:** strengthens the Kidneys.

✓ **Walnuts and walnut oil:** nourish Kidney *Yang* and strengthen the Lungs.

✓ **Warming, cooked foods.**

Liver Qi stagnation

- Asthma symptoms.
- Muscle tension.
- Tightness in the chest.
- Worse with emotional upset.
- Triggered by an allergen.

This type of asthma is usually seen in older children over the age of seven. Dietary advice for asthma should be followed. Figuring out what the allergens are through testing will be helpful to reduce exposure when beginning treatment. Stress reduction techniques, such as yoga, guided meditations, and deep breathing exercises, are all indicated.

DIETARY THERAPY

✓ All the above **dietary recommendations for asthma** should be followed.

✓ **Lighter meals:** diet consists mainly of fruit, vegetables, and whole grains.

✓ **Combine rich foods**, like meat, with greens or low-starch vegetables, like asparagus, broccoli, cauliflower, cabbage, cucumber, peppers, and celery.

✓ **Cabbage (red and green):** neutral to warming; regulates *Qi*.

✓ **Chives:** warming, pungent, slightly bitter.

✓ **Celery:** benefits the Liver and clears heat.

✓ **Dried orange peel** (can be dried from an unsprayed mandarin or tangerine and steeped into a tea): dries dampness and transforms phlegm. Moves *Qi*.

- ✓ **Fennel:** warming, pungent, sweet; spreads Liver *Qi*, warms Kidney *Yang*.
- ✓ **Green bell peppers:** cooling, pungent, bitter; move *Qi*.
- ✓ **Leeks:** warming, pungent, sweet; move *Qi*.
- ✓ **Onions:** warming, pungent, sweet; move *Qi*.
- ✓ **Sour flavor:** a little sour flavor in the diet will help to move Liver *Qi*, such as lemon or lime squeezed into water, or vinegar used in sauces and cooking. Sourdough breads are also great.
- ✓ **Spices:** incorporate lots of bitter and pungent spices: fennel seed, turmeric, basil, bay leaf, caraway seed, cardamom, mint, coriander, rosemary, and paprika.

Bedwetting (nocturnal enuresis)

When a child is frequently unable to control their bladder at night, it can be a disturbing and disruptive time for families. I remember a mom, whose child had nocturnal enuresis, recounting her tip on how she managed the nights: layer the bed with three layers of sheets—a sheet protector, then a regular sheet, then another sheet protector followed by another regular sheet, followed by another sheet protector and regular sheet! This way she could easily peel off the soiled layer without having to remake the bed—a great solution for getting back to sleep quickly, but not for the enuresis. Children can have occasional instances of wetting the bed up until the age of seven; it is when bedwetting occurs on a regular basis (once or twice a week for months on end) that it requires treatment. A pediatrician or doctor can rule out any underlying medical conditions. TCM recognizes that there is almost always an underlying Kidney deficiency in a child who is bedwetting as the Kidneys control the flow of Body Fluids in the Lower Burner (Kidney, Bladder, Large Intestine, and Small Intestine) and the balance between Kidney *Yin* and *Yang* controls the lower "gate" of urination. For this reason, the diet should include foods that nourish the Kidneys and then also include either Spleen- and Lung-nourishing foods or foods that will help to eliminate damp-heat. Constipation has been indicated as one of the reasons that could cause bedwetting in children (Hodges *et al.* 2012; Hsiao *et al.* 2020). Making sure that children's bowels are moving regularly is an important factor in maintaining a healthy baseline.

Kidney deficiency

- Nocturnal enuresis 1–2 times per evening.
- Larger amount of urine.
- Frequent urination throughout the day.
- Easy to fatigue.

DIETARY THERAPY

- ✓ Traditionally **wheat berries** (whole grain form of wheat) have been used in TCM to help with bedwetting. Wheat berries have a cooling thermal nature, are sweet and salty in nature, strengthen the Kidneys, mildly astringe the *Yin*, and nourish and calm the heart-mind (see following page for **Popped Wheat Berries**).
- ✓ **Black Bean Aquafaba:** helps with bedwetting. Black beans are warming and tonify the Kidneys You can utilize the thick water drained from a can of black beans (or see below for a recipe).
- ✓ **Black sesame seeds:** nourish Kidney *Yin*.
- ✓ **Bone broths:** the minerals nourish the Kidneys deeply.
- ✓ **Eggs:** nourish Kidney *Jing*.
- ✓ **Goat milk:** nourishes Kidney *Jing* and Kidney *Yang*.
- ✓ **Lentils:** nourish Kidney *Jing*.
- ✓ **Millet:** tonifies Kidney *Yin*.
- ✓ **Quinoa:** tonifies Kidney *Yang*.
- ✓ **Walnuts and walnut oil:** nourish Kidney *Yang*.

Avoid or eliminate:

- + Cold, chilled, or iced food or drink.
- + Raw food.

BLACK BEAN AQUAFABA
Ingredients
- 1 cup of black beans covered in water and soaked overnight
- 6 cups of water

Method
1. Drain the soaking water from the beans and rinse them under water.
2. Add the beans and 6 cups of water to a pot and bring to a boil.
3. Reduce the heat and simmer for one hour. After one hour, check if

beans are done (soft enough). If they need more time, check them in 15-minute intervals.

4. When done, drain the liquid from the beans, reserving it.
5. If the child dislikes the flavor, add the "juice" to a soup or make into a miso soup. Drink ½ cup twice daily. Beans can be eaten.

POPPED WHEAT BERRIES

These can be added to cereals, porridges, salads, enjoyed with non-dairy milk poured over, or eaten by the handful.

Ingredients
- ½ cup of wheat berries, uncooked
- 1 tsp oil
- Salt to taste

Method
1. Heat a cast-iron or heavy-bottomed saucepan to a medium to high heat.
2. When the saucepan is sizzling hot, add the oil.
3. Add the wheat berries and stir constantly for about 3 minutes until done. Make in batches of ½ cup at a time. They will be done when they are easy to eat with a crunch. Watch they do not burn.
4. Remove from the saucepan and add salt to taste.

Spleen and Lung Qi deficiency

- Nocturnal enuresis happens periodically, especially post-illness or when fatigued.
- Small amount of urine with bedwetting and a little amount of urination throughout the day (but may be frequent).
- Pale face.
- Loose stools.
- Easily catches colds and coughs.
- Low appetite.

DIETARY THERAPY

✓ **Spleen Qi nourishing diet.**

✓ **Almonds:** benefit the Lungs; can use almond milk.

✓ **Apples:** benefit the Lungs.

✓ **Apricots (dried or fresh):** neutral thermal nature; enter the Lungs and benefit the Lungs.

✓ **Pears:** benefit the Lungs.

✓ **Walnuts and walnut oil:** benefit both the Lungs and Kidneys.

+ Reduce sugar intake.

Avoid or eliminate:

+ Cold, chilled, or iced food or drink.

+ Raw food.

Damp-heat

• Urine that has a strong smell.

• Burning urination.

• Irritability.

DIETARY THERAPY

✓ **Adzuki/red beans:** neutral thermal nature; drain dampness and tonify the Kidneys.

✓ **Celery:** cooling thermal nature; relieves dampness and cools the Liver.

✓ **Dark leafy greens:** generally cooling and bitter, which drains damp-heat.

✓ **Mung beans:** cooling thermal nature; reduce damp-heat conditions in the body.

✓ **Rye:** neutral thermal nature; drains dampness, moves Liver *Qi*.

+ Reduce intake of nut butters.

Avoid or eliminate:

+ Fatty, greasy, and fried foods.

+ Spicy foods.

+ Sugar and sweets.

Colic

Parents of newborns will want to know how to help their baby if they start to show signs of colic. Not knowing what to do can feel stressful when a little baby is crying for hours on end each day, for seemingly no reason. They are fed, napped, snuggled, and diaper changed; all the boxes have been ticked for what would normally cause a baby to cry. Colic typically begins in the first month of life and will end by around three to four months on its own. It is essentially indigestion causing pain and discomfort due to excess gas and bloating. The crying usually occurs in the late afternoon and evening and the babies may pump their legs towards their bellies. They are unable to properly digest the milk they are being fed, or might be feeding too frequently, which then causes food stagnation (accumulation disorder) in the digestive tract. They will sometimes stop crying when they are able to pass gas. The root is Spleen *Qi* deficiency and a baby may present with either hot- or cold-type colic. With a few changes to the feeding schedule, a little help from fennel, and an abdominal massage, the colic should resolve quickly.

Hot-type colic

- Red face.
- Feels hot to touch.
- Excess gas.
- Smelly stools.
- Restless.
- Strong cry.
- More common than cold-type colic.

DIETARY THERAPY

When a baby has colic (or even for prevention) it is necessary for the mother to try and establish a regular feeding schedule instead of feeding on demand. For the first month of life it *is* recommended to feed a newborn on demand to keep the milk supply up and because newborns are often hungry. After this first month, though, nursing between seven to nine times per day is optimal. This way it is less likely that the baby will overfeed, causing stagnation in the Stomach and Intestines, leading to heat accumulation.

- ✓ **Space between feeds**, to allow more time for the baby to digest milk.
- ✓ **Massage the baby's lower abdomen:** starting in the lower right side of the abdomen, go up, then left across the top, and downwards on

the left side of the abdomen, then back to the start on the right side, moving in a clockwise direction, following the route of the large intestine (ascending colon on the right and descending on the left). You can use the flat fingertips of your dominant hand using small clockwise circles as the large intestine is traced.

✓ Give 1 tsp of **Fennel Seed and Lemon Balm Tea** (see below) to the baby three times daily. If the breastfeeding mother drinks a few cups of this tea daily, the benefits will pass along through the breast milk. The mother may also drink chamomile or dill seed tea. Fennel seed is warming and stimulates digestion. Lemon balm is cooling and helps to relieve gas.

✓ **Mother's diet:** the mother may need to reduce caffeine, sugar, garlic, onion, Brussels sprouts, cauliflower, broccoli, cabbage, tomatoes, citrus foods, and dairy.

✓ If the baby is on formula, the parents may need to try switching from a cow's milk base to a **goat milk-based formula** to help with digestion.

✓ In *The Nourishing Traditions Book of Baby and Child Care*, Sally Fallon Morell and Thomas S. Cowan suggest that a mother may have an overabundance of milk, and that if this is the case, the baby "may end up getting too much foremilk, which is rich in lactose, and not enough hindmilk, which is rich in fat. The overabundance of lactose may be hard for baby to digest, leading to gas and fussiness; and the lack of fat may lead to low blood sugar, crankiness, and the need to nurse more frequently. The solution is to give one breast only during a feeding so that it is emptied completely" (2013, p.137).

FENNEL SEED AND LEMON BALM TEA
Ingredients
- 1 organic fennel teabag or 1 tsp fennel seeds
- 1 organic lemon balm teabag or 1½ tsp dried lemon balm or 1 tbsp fresh lemon balm leaves
- 2 cups of hot water

Method
1. Steep the herbs in hot water for 10 minutes.
2. Strain and allow to cool completely before serving.

Cold-type colic

- Pale face.
- Blue vein on the bridge of the nose.
- Cold hands and feet.
- Cry lacks force.

With the deficient form of colic, Spleen *Qi* deficiency is at the root of the stagnation. Overfeeding needs to be addressed to prevent the already deficient weak Spleen energy from further damage.

DIETARY THERAPY

- ✓ **Space between feeds** to avoid overworking the Spleen.
- ✓ Follow all the same advice as for hot-type colic but *instead:* **massage the lower abdomen** along the same route of the large intestine, but the *small circles* need to be massaged *counter*clockwise.
- ✓ Give 1 tsp **Fennel Seed and Lemon Balm Tea** (see above) three times a day along with a few drops of **Fennel and Ginger Juice Tea** (see below). Fennel is warming and stimulates digestion. Ginger is warming, circulates *Qi*, and warms the digestion.

FENNEL AND GINGER JUICE TEA
Ingredients
- 1 organic fennel teabag or 1 tsp fennel seeds
- 1 thumb-sized piece of raw ginger

Method
1. Steep the fennel in hot water for 10 minutes.
2. Strain and allow to cool.
3. In the meantime, peel the raw ginger, place in a blender and blend.
4. Once the ginger has broken down, use a cheesecloth or press through a tea strainer to extract any juice.
5. Place a few drops of ginger juice in each dose of fennel tea given to the baby: dosage of tea is 1 tsp, three times daily.

Stomach ache

Stomach aches are quite common in children. They can be fleeting, arising suddenly in the mornings, and gone an hour later. Oftentimes, younger children have not yet connected what the feeling of having to "go number two" feels like, and will only know it as a stomach ache. Encouraging the child to try going to the bathroom may be all that is required to relieve the pain. Stomach aches can be a physical manifestation of anxiety. If they happen frequently, find out if they always occur before school or an afterschool activity or even when the parent has to leave for work—any situation that could be causing anxiety in the child. Even when the pain is due to anxiety, it is real to the child, and it can be reassuring for them to know that there is something they can eat to help relieve the pain. A warming heat pack on their abdomen can be very soothing. Stomach aches can be due to either sudden cold attacks, a result of deficiency, retention of food, or from phlegm accumulation (discussed under "Vomit" later).

Candied Ginger (see below) is a wonderful remedy to have on hand for all of these etiologies. Ginger is warming, strengthens the Middle Burner, transforms phlegm, and promotes digestion. It's easy to pack along to have on hand when needed. The sweet flavor also helps to harmonize pain.

CANDIED GINGER

Ingredients

- 3 cups of ginger, sliced ⅛ inch thick (either thinly slice with a knife or use a mandolin)
- Pinch of salt
- 2 cups of raw cane sugar (or evaporated cane sugar)

Method

1. Place the ginger in a saucepan and cover with water.
2. Bring to a boil, then reduce and simmer for 30 minutes.
3. Reserve ½ cup of the water and drain the rest (or keep and drink).
4. Place the drained ginger back into the pan with the reserved water, a pinch of salt and the sugar.
5. Bring to a boil, reduce the heat to medium, stir frequently, and simmer until the sugar syrup seems dry, has almost evaporated, and starts to recrystallize—about 20 minutes (or until a candy thermometer reads 225°F).

6. Drain the ginger over a bowl to save the syrup (which is great for making into a drink).
7. Lay the ginger on a cooling rack over a pan that can catch the drippings, and let it completely dry (ideally overnight).
8. This will keep for several months in an airtight container.

Cold in the Middle Burner

- Severe, sudden onset, which can be relieved by warmth; aggravated by pressure.
- Pain brought on after eating cold-natured foods or from exposing abdominal area to exterior cold.
- Pale face.
- Sweating.
- Cold limbs.

DIETARY THERAPY

- ✓ **Warming, cooked foods.**
- ✓ **Cardamom:** disperses cold. Can open the pod and eat the seed, a few pieces at a time, or sprinkle the powder onto oatmeal or smoothies.
- ✓ **Fennel:** warm and pungent, affects the stomach. Can use with ginger as a seasoning for cooking.
- ✓ **Ginger:** warms the Middle Burner.
- ✓ **Honey:** helps to relieve pain. Dissolve a few tablespoons in warm water and drink once a day.

Until there is improvement, no:

+ Raw foods.
+ Bananas, tomatoes, avocado, or oranges.
+ Chilled, iced, or frozen food and drink.

Spleen Qi and or Yang deficiency

- Dull pain relieved by pressure and food intake.
- Pale complexion.
- Diarrhea or loose stools with undigested food.

- Cold limbs.
- Low appetite.
- Bloating after eating.

DIETARY THERAPY

All of the above spices used for excess cold can also be used here. This syndrome will come and go and will require longer-term dietary shifts. Nourishing the Spleen *Qi* is a must, and the reduction of raw and cold foods must be for the longer term.

Food stagnation (retention of food)

- Abdominal distention.
- Bad breath (we call it "kitten breath" in our family!).
- Low appetite.
- Diarrhea or vomit relieved by bowel movement.

Any time there is an accumulation of food it must be dispersed to relieve the pain. If the child has Spleen *Qi* deficiency signs, the long-term diet must support this.

DIETARY THERAPY

- ✓ **Coriander:** warming and pungent. Breaks down and moves food accumulation.
- ✓ **Hawthorn berries:** relieve food stagnation, especially from meat and dairy. Can be eaten raw if found locally (but need to spit out the seeds), or dried berries can be ordered online or found at health food stores and brewed into tea.
- ✓ **Marjoram:** cooling and pungent. Promotes digestion, moves *Qi*.
- ✓ **Radish seeds:** can be found more easily in Asian food markets. They can be crushed to create a juice and added to water.
- ✓ **Sprouted barley:** used to relieve food stagnation, especially if it is from grains. Can use the sweetener made from sprouted barley called **malted barley**, a little dissolved into warm water. Coffee substitutes such as Bambu® will often contain malted barley. These are great to keep on hand and need only be dissolved into hot water to drink; they can be lightly sweetened for children.
- ✓ **Sprouted rice and millet grains** are used for food stagnation. It does

take a few days to sprout the grain, though, in which case the food stagnation may have passed. Some stores now carry sprouted grains.

✓ **Combine aniseed, fennel, caraway and cumin seeds** into a bowl and nibble on a teaspoon of the mixture after meals, to aid digestion.

+ Watch for overeating or overfeeding.

Nausea and vomit

Nausea and vomit are common in younger children as the Spleen and Stomach are immature and sometimes cannot digest food properly. A little bit of spitting up is normal in a baby, especially in the first three months of life. It is a problem if it becomes vomit, when the spitting up is actually forceful and shoots out a few inches.

Vomit due to a viral stomach infection or food poisoning is best helped by our old friend, ginger. Sipping small sips of **Ginger Tea or Soda** will aid the stomach *Qi* to go back down instead of up, and is also indicated to alleviate vomit.

GINGER TEA OR SODA

Ingredients
- 4–5 thumb-sized pieces of ginger root (you can leave the peel on)
- 2 cups of water

Method
1. Place the ginger root into soda water and let sit for 5 minutes before serving.
2. To make tea, place the ginger and water into a saucepan and bring to a boil.
3. Reduce the heat and simmer for 10 minutes. Strain the ginger and serve.

Retention of food

If this condition does not resolve, it can lead to accumulation disorder.

- Sour-smelling vomit.
- Can happen because of overeating or eating difficult to digest foods (a day at the amusement park!).
- Restlessness.

✓ **Ginger is the best remedy.** It will harmonize the Stomach and descend Stomach *Qi*.

✓ **Coriander:** warming and pungent. Breaks down and moves food accumulation.

✓ **Hawthorn berries:** relieve food stagnation, especially from meat and dairy. Can be eaten raw if found locally (but need to spit out the seeds), or dried berries can be ordered online or found at health food stores and brewed into tea.

✓ **Marjoram:** cooling and pungent. Promotes digestion, moves *Qi*.

✓ **Radish seeds:** can be found more easily in Asian food markets. They can be crushed to create a juice and added to water.

✓ **Sprouted barley:** used to relieve food stagnation, especially if it is from grains. Can use the sweetener made from sprouted barley called **malted barley**, a little dissolved into warm water. Coffee substitutes such as Bambu® will often contain malted barley. These are great to keep on hand and need only be dissolved into hot water to drink; they can be lightly sweetened for children.

✓ **Sprouted rice and millet grains** are used for food stagnation. It does take a few days to sprout the grain, though, in which case the food stagnation may have passed. Some stores now carry sprouted grains.

✓ **Combine aniseed, fennel, caraway and cumin seeds** into a bowl and nibble on a teaspoon of the mixture after meals, to aid digestion.

+ Watch for overeating or overfeeding.
+ No greasy, difficult-to-digest foods.

Spleen and Stomach deficiency

- Vomit contains undigested food.
- Vomit has little odor.
- Vomit may be clear fluid and a small amount.
- Low appetite.
- Pale face.
- With phlegm involvement, the child will vomit phlegm or a clear, sticky fluid. Happens occasionally and they may have other signs of phlegm, such as congestion in the chest or sinuses.

As the root of the problem is Spleen and Stomach deficiency, this will need to be addressed with a Spleen *Qi* nourishing diet for overall health. There is usually cold in the Stomach in this condition, so warming the Stomach is indicated. With phlegm involvement, phlegm should be transformed.

DIETARY THERAPY

- ✓ **Ginger is the best remedy.** It will harmonize the stomach and descend Stomach *Qi*. Can make a **Ginger and Rice Congee** (see below) as this is easy to digest.
- ✓ **Spleen *Qi* nourishing diet.**
- ✓ **Caraway seed:** warming and pungent, indicated for vomit.
- ✓ **Cardamom:** warming and pungent, indicated for vomit.
- ✓ **Non-caffeinated Chai tea:** steep the tea and allow the child to drink a few sips at a time. Chai teas usually contain a blend of spices helpful for vomit, including cardamom, black pepper, and cloves.
- ✓ **Cloves:** warming and pungent, and push the energy downward. Affect the Stomach and indicated for Stomach cold vomiting.
- ✓ **Fennel:** warming and pungent, and affects the Stomach.
- ✓ **Nutmeg:** warming and pungent, and pushes the energy downward.

GINGER AND RICE CONGEE
Ingredients
- ½ cup of uncooked rice
- 3 x 1-inch slices of ginger
- 3 cups of water
- 1 tbsp oil
- 1 tbsp tamari
- 4 cups of stock (chicken or vegetable)

Method
1. Combine the rice, water and oil in a bowl and let soak for 1–2 hours (you can skip the soaking step if there is not enough time).
2. When ready to cook, add the stock, ginger, tamari, and rice to a saucepan.
3. Bring to a boil over a medium to high heat.
4. Reduce the heat to a simmer and cover the pan, leaving a small gap.
5. Simmer for 1 hour and 15 minutes. Stir occasionally to prevent the rice sticking to the bottom.
6. Remove the ginger pieces before serving.

With phlegm involvement, add the following:

- ✓ **Mustard seeds:** warm and pungent, and resolve phlegm.
- ✓ **Dried citrus peel** (can make at home with unsprayed tangerine or mandarin orange peel): warming, transforms phlegm, and harmonizes the Middle Burner.

Ear infections

Ear infections are common in children—most will experience at least one ear infection before the age of seven. The Western medicine treatment method is currently a "watchful waiting" approach, and if that doesn't work, antibiotics are then prescribed. Eighty percent of ear infections do resolve on their own in a few days (they are often viral in nature), and pain management is the best treatment method (Venekamp, Damoiseaux, and Schilder 2014). This "watchful waiting" approach prevents the antibiotics cycle that can occur when antibiotics are needlessly used. Antibiotics are cold in nature and will clear heat, thus achieving pain relief, but they can also damage Spleen and Stomach *Qi*, further exacerbating the potential root condition. One of the reasons for ear infections in children is due to stagnant food accumulating in the Stomach and Intestines. This causes heat to rise along the internal pathway that connects the Stomach and Intestines to the inner ear. This is often seen in children who are teething or when solid foods are first introduced, causing digestive difficulty. If the ear infection is due to an exterior pathogenic factor, combine the dietary indications for an exterior pathogenic factor with the treatment methods below.

Symptoms include:

- Acts fussy (babies or young children); is grumpy.
- Pulls at ears.
- May have a fever.

DIETARY THERAPY

- ✓ **Bland diet.**
- ✓ **Spleen *Qi* nourishing diet.**

External poultice: Cut an onion in half. Warm slightly with the cut side down in a saucepan. Make sure it is not too hot before placing over the sore ear. Hold on the ear for 5–10 minutes, also placing on the area behind the earlobe. Treat both ears the same way.

+ Watch for overeating or overfeeding.

Reduce or eliminate:

+ Cold, chilled, or iced food or drink.
+ Dairy.
+ Greasy, fatty, or fried foods.
+ Ice cream, popsicles.
+ Sugar.

Low appetite

Children's appetites can vary greatly; they can go months with extraordinarily little appetite and occasionally may even refuse to eat, and then suddenly they start asking for more food. Appetite levels can correlate with growth and activity. Even when eating little, children can be full of energy and spirit. There are many different psychological reasons for either refusing to eat or eating only one type of food or not showing much interest in food. For the root condition to be treated, these psychological factors need to be taken into consideration. For the purposes of dietary therapy, I list foods that stimulate the appetite that can be used as an adjunct to any other treatments being utilized.

DIETARY THERAPY

✓ **Dill:** warming and pungent, helps appetite.
✓ **Dried citrus peel brewed as tea** (can make at home with unsprayed tangerine or mandarin orange peel): warming, and is indicated for lack of appetite.
✓ **Figs:** neutral thermal nature; strengthen the Spleen and harmonize the Stomach; indicated for lack of appetite and indigestion.
✓ **Lotus seeds:** neutral thermal nature; nourish the Spleen; indicated for loss of appetite.

Food stagnation

* Low appetite.
* Does not want to eat or drink.
* Bloated abdomen.
* Flatulence.
* Bad breath.

- ✓ **All the recommendations above to improve appetite.**
- ✓ **Coriander:** warming and pungent. Breaks down and moves food accumulation.
- ✓ **Hawthorn berries:** relieve food stagnation, especially from meat and dairy. Can be eaten raw if found locally (but need to spit out the seeds), or dried berries can be ordered online or found at health food stores and brewed into tea.
- ✓ **Marjoram:** cooling and pungent. Promotes digestion, moves *Qi*.
- ✓ **Sprouted rice and millet grains** are used for food stagnation. It does take a few days to sprout the grain, though, in which case the food stagnation may have passed. Some stores now carry sprouted grains.
- ✓ **Radish seeds:** can be found more easily in Asian food markets. They can be crushed to create a juice and added to water.
- ✓ **Sprouted barley:** used to relieve food stagnation, especially if it is from grains. Can use the sweetener made from sprouted barley called **malted barley**, a little dissolved into warm water. Coffee substitutes such as Bambu® will often contain malted barley. These are great to keep on hand and need only be dissolved into hot water to drink; they can be lightly sweetened for children.
- ✓ **Combine aniseed, fennel, caraway and cumin seeds** into a bowl and nibble on a teaspoon of the mixture after meals, to aid digestion.
- ✓ **Massage the abdomen** in a clockwise direction.

- + Watch for overeating.

Spleen and Stomach Qi deficiency

- Low appetite.
- Fatigue.
- May have loose stools with undigested food.
- Pale face.

- ✓ **Spleen *Qi* nourishing diet.**
- ✓ **All the recommendations to improve appetite.**

Reduce or eliminate:

+ Chilled, frozen, or iced food and drink.
+ Raw food.
+ Sugar.

A few extras

Burns: Apply honey directly to the burn. Research shows this to be an effective treatment as honey has anti-infectious, anti-inflammatory, anti-exudative, antioxidant, wound healing, wound debriding, and nutritional properties (Zbuchea 2014).

Swallowing a metallic object: From Paul Pitchford, *Healing with Whole Foods*: "If a child swallows a metallic object such as a coin, feed him plenty of sweet potato, which will stick to the object and allow it to come out easier in the feces" (2002, p.550). I don't know anyone who has tried this, but it sounds like it would work wonderfully!

Wasp or bee sting: Use the poultice of a fresh onion. Slice an onion in half and place it flesh side down over the sting until the pain starts to subside.

CHAPTER 10

The Tao of Food Positivity

The ancient mothers knew.
 There was no need for books and experts.
 Today we have lost much.
 We need to relearn the Way.
 Be cautious about what the experts tell you.
 What sounds complex and clever may have no roots. Wisdom has
no cleverness in it.
 It is pure and simple, and when it is practiced the results are obvious.
 The wise assist a child's being rather than his doing.

McClure (1997, p.116)

Our memories and experiences connected to meals and eating can take us back to childhood. I can still conjure up the sight and taste of my grandmother's freshly baked carrot cake she would make whenever the family connected for meals. Perfectly moist and delicious, we always looked forward to it! There were also times when I can remember dreading dinner due to feeling full and knowing I would still be made to eat more food. I think we are all familiar with the phrases "You are not leaving the table until you have finished your plate" or "No dessert until you have eaten your dinner." These power struggles do not need to happen for children to be eating enough.

Food therapy for children encompasses so much more than writing out a list of foods to help with an ailment. Eating together as a family daily, celebrating occasions with special meals served around the table, viewing the dinner table as a sacred space where communication is focused on pleasing conversation, and minimizing eating on the run—these are all important factors to fostering positive experiences around eating and mealtimes.

Jamie Oliver, a well-known chef and advocate for healthy eating and reducing childhood obesity, expressed this beautifully in his 2010 Ted Talk "Teach every child about food:" "I profoundly believe that the power of food has a primal place in our homes, that binds us to the best bits of life."[1]

The more experiences children have around meals and food that are positive, the better equipped they will be as teenagers and young adults to create healthy habits for themselves. It has been shown that regular meals eaten together as a family evolved into long-term beneficial influences on children's biopsychosocial wellbeing by age 10, such as lower levels of soft drink consumption, physical aggression, oppositional behavior, non-aggressive delinquency, and reactive regression (Harbec and Pagani 2018).

Positive experiences around food will also foster the parent–child attachment as it aims to eliminate strife and discord pertaining to food and eating. On the school grounds during afterschool pickup I have observed parents checking children's lunch bags to see if their contents have been eaten, and then admonishing the child if much has been left untouched. Battles over how much and what is eaten can, over time, fuel resentment, refusal to eat, or ingrain the message that continuing to eat past fullness is normal. This all comes from a place of love as parents genuinely worry their children are not eating enough or obtaining proper nutrition. I have been guilty of all the above at one time or another. It takes practice to let go of control and trust in the innate knowledge a child's growing body has in regard to how much they require at different times and that, if given healthy choices, they will get all they need to grow healthy and strong.

In the 1920s, Clare M. Davis, a pediatrician from Chicago in the USA, asked the question, "What will babies eat if they're given free choice?" To answer this, she observed 15 children over six years in an orphanage (Davis 1939). The children were between the ages of 6 and 11 months old. No child could stay in the study for longer than two-and-a-half years. Since they were close to or had just been weaned, they hadn't had a chance to develop food preferences (although we now know the amniotic fluid surrounding a fetus contains many flavors from the maternal diet, and babies will show preferences for food their mothers ate; see Mennella *et al.* 2001). Nonetheless, 33 different types of food were offered each day, split up into three meals, in different bowls, and set before the child. Nurses were then instructed to only feed the items that the children either pointed at or grabbed on their own without showing any facial expressions or making comments that might imply a choice was good or bad. There was none of the

---

1   www.ted.com/talks/jamie_oliver_teach_every_child_about_food?language=en

sort of junk food, processed, sugary stuff that is marketed at kids today. A selection of the foods up for offer were water, sweet milk, sour milk, sea salt, apples, orange juice, tomatoes, beets, potatoes, turnips, cauliflower, cabbage, wheat, oatmeal, barley, beef, bone marrow, chicken, sweetbreads, liver, and fish. The children could eat as much or as little as they chose, and whichever kinds of foods they wanted, without any interference, guidance, or force-feeding. When the child stopped eating, the tray was taken away. Clare found that of the 15 different babies, 15 different eating patterns emerged. The foods they chose were unusual (as we see it) for that age group. Some would choose liver and orange juice for breakfast and then have several eggs, bananas, and milk for supper. Dieticians would weigh the dishes before and after each meal, even taking into account food spilled on to the ground. Despite the varied, random, and self-selected nature of foods, all the babies met their normal caloric and nutritional needs for their age group; they had lots of energy for playing and they thrived. Some of the infants received for the study had started out in poor condition; they were poorly nourished and underweight, and a few had rickets. One child with severe rickets was given a small glass of cod liver oil on his tray for him to take if he chose. This he did irregularly and in varying amounts until his blood calcium and phosphorus became normal and X-ray film showed his rickets to be healed, after which he did not take it again.

The consensus among doctors at the time this study took place was to give strict instructions to parents about not only the types but also the quantities of food. This created a counter-will in many children who then refused to eat at all. Davis believed that the children's erratic way of eating—wanting to eat breakfast one day but not the next, enjoying chicken for a while then not, licking their plates clean one evening but barely touching their food another—was completely normal and should be afforded.

The fact that all 15 children in the study could eat a widely different assortment of fruits, vegetables, meat, and grains and all achieve uniform health and nutritional balance was concluded by Davis to be "wisdom of the body": "Such successful juggling and balancing of the more than 30 nutritional essentials that exist in mixed and different proportions in the foods from which they must be derived suggests at once the existence of some innate, automatic mechanism for its accomplishment" (quoted in Strauss 2006). They could have easily avoided a major food group and developed anemia, scurvy, or not healed from the rickets, but all the children had hearty appetites, healthy immune systems, none had constipation, and colds were the mild, three-day type.

An important caveat to consider with this study is the nature of the food that was offered—wholesome, seasonal, and locally available fruits and vegetables—with the omission of salt-laden, processed, and sugary fare. Davis herself concluded that the selection of food for children should be left "in the hands of their elders where everyone has always known it belongs" (quoted in Strauss 2006). Davis was planning on conducting a different version of the study—she wanted to know what would happen if, alongside the plethora of healthy food that she had offered the children, candy bars, cakes, and chips were also on the menu. Would the infants still have the innate ability to acquire all the necessary nutrition to grow healthy, or would the empty calories interfere with the process? Suffice to say, we could see the outcome for the children would not have been as health-giving as the first experiment. The Great Depression dashed her hopes of ever finding out for certain, and no later studies of the same nature were conducted due to the ethical and moral implications involved in such research. Her seminal work is widely understood to be an important factor in lifelong healthy eating habits and is now seen as a means of reducing adult obesity.

Fast-forward to 2020, a newly released scientific statement from the American Heart Association (AHA) published evidence-based strategies for caregivers on how to create a healthy food environment. Their conclusions—identical to what Claire Davis had discovered in the 1920s and what the very core of Taoist food philosophy embodies—allow children to choose what and how much to eat and not to feel pressured by their caregiver's wishes and demands during mealtime within an environment composed of healthy, seasonal, and balanced choices. The research showed that this encouraged ownership over their decisions about food and may help them develop eating patterns linked to a healthy weight for a lifetime. "Parents and caregivers should consider building a positive food environment centered on healthy eating habits, rather than focusing on rigid rules about what and how a child should eat," says Alexis C. Wood, the writing group chair for the AHA Scientific Statement and Assistant Professor at the US Department of Agriculture/Agriculture Research Services Children's Nutrition Research Center and the Department of Pediatrics (Nutrition section) at Baylor College of Medicine in Houston (Wood *et al.* 2020).[2]

The other added bonus of letting go of the control over exactly what and how much children are made to eat will eliminate tension and battles

---

2   See https://newsroom.heart.org/news/healthy-eating-behaviors-in-childhood-may-reduce-the-risk-of-adult-obesity-and-heart-disease?preview=6808

over lunches left uneaten, picked-over dinners, and days when it seems as if birds eat more than they do. But then when they suddenly eat their plate clean of Brussels sprouts, tofu, and a quinoa vegetable medley, parents can breathe a sigh of relief—their little bodies can be trusted to know what is required and when. As quoted from the *Tao Te Ching* (Lao Tzu translation by Stephen Mitchell),

Therefore the Master (essentially us)
acts without doing anything
and teaches without saying anything.

The recommendations below will help families incorporate positivity surrounding their children's diets that is backed by research and aims to foster an appreciation for healthy food, self-regulation in regard to nutritional needs, and to strengthen the parent–child relationship. It should be noted that if there are special circumstances such as childhood diseases or disorders, issues with weight gain, refusal to eat, or any circumstances surrounding a child's diet that are abnormal, a referral to a pediatrician is recommended.

Strive for peaceful mealtimes and a time for connection: This is like the cherry on the cake. If a lot of consideration has gone into creating a nourishing, seasonal, health-promoting meal, it only makes sense to create an atmosphere that will foster optimal digestion. Stress while eating puts bodies into fight or flight mode, which then takes priority away from digestion: blood is diverted from the organs to the limbs to get the body ready to RUN! In TCM we know that stress (Liver *Qi*) attacks the digestion (Spleen *Qi*) and over time weakens the Spleen *Qi* and causes problems such as constipation, nausea, stomach ache, and loose stools. Conflict-free conversation, no distractions (phones, television, books) and not rushing will all contribute to less stress at the table. Focusing on the meal instead of reading or watching something else is a helpful habit to promote.

Offer an assortment of healthy food options for breakfast, lunch, and dinner, and resist the urge to comment on what a child has or has not consumed: Children eat naturally and spontaneously. Offer meals with no strings attached. Let go of any expectation as to the outcome of what or how much is eaten. Applauding a meal left uneaten would not occur to us, as grateful as we should be that a child has self-regulated their appetite. It's helpful to introduce new foods regularly alongside foods they enjoy. Frequent exposure to new foods has been found to increase the likelihood of children eventually eating them (Zeinstra, Vrijhof, and Kremer 2018). Even if children don't eat the vegetables on their plates the first time, they might the 10th or 15th time! Taking a back-seat approach to mealtimes may even help to prevent adult obesity and heart disease (AHA 2020).

Practice mindfulness at meals: Children are naturals at mindful eating. They can take a morsel of food, smell it, study it, turn it over, lick it, smell it again, tear it apart, smell it again, slowly take a little bite, chew it 30 times, all the while focusing solely on this one little morsel of food. It can drive an adult crazy watching this and wishing they would hurry up and eat. Incorporating some mindfulness techniques in conjunction with eating will bring awareness to appetite, how the food got to the table, gratitude for the abundance we have, and greater enjoyment of food. A mindful eating technique that can be turned into a fun game is to use an almond or a strawberry, for example, and first ask the child to check in to how their body is feeling—are they hungry, not hungry, is their tummy grumbling? Then ask the child to look closely at the food, investigating its texture, color, and smell. Really look at and notice the food. Then, ask them to place it in the mouth, take some time to appreciate how it feels on the tongue, and start chewing, taking the time to chew it as much as possible, noticing how the flavor changes the longer it is held in the mouth. With younger children this mindful practice can start with simple questions for them, such as, "What color is the strawberry?", "Does it have seeds in it?", or "Does the strawberry feel soft or hard?"

To cultivate a mindful eating practice with children:

- Focus the attention on everyone who is at the table. This would mean no electronic devices, books, or toys that could pose a distraction.
- Tune in to appetite level.
- Express gratitude for the food and all the work and energy required along the food chain to get it to the plate.
- Talk about the different foods on the plate, the seasonality of the ingredients, how the food is grown, ways it can be eaten, and the ethnicity of the cuisine, if applicable.
- Notice how the body and mind feels after eating—happier, less tired, more tired, content, craving anything, feeling full, or any digestive discomfort.

Gratitude: A study conducted in Japan with school children found a connection between appreciating food and what children ate for lunch (Akamatsu *et al.* 2019). All children in Japan eat the same lunch cooked at the school with a daily changing menu. It is my dream to bring this same model to Canada. Students are involved, on a rotating basis, in cooking, serving, and cleaning up the meal, served to every student. Lunches are healthy and part of the school's health education program. The study from Akamatsu *et al.* (2019) was conducted with 662 students, asking them to respond to statements using a five-point Likert scale. Some of the statements in the study included were: "I am thankful for the food that gave us its life," "I am thankful for the people who grew the food and cooked the school lunch," and "I care about the seasonality of the food I eat for school lunch." They found that having school dieticians teach the students gratitude for the food and the people involved in food production helped to decrease food dislikes among children, promoted greater enjoyment of eating, and reduced food waste.

Giving thanks does not require a religious connotation. Simply appreciating the effort and hard work that took place along the way to get food to the plate that is about to be eaten is also a great mindfulness practice—thank you to the seeds, sun, rain, animals, farmers, store employees, etc., anyone or anything that played a part in getting the meal to the table.

Resist the temptation to use sweet food as a "reward," a "treat," or as a "bribe": "Sugar is not love. But it can feel like it" (Wilson 2015, p.17). This quote from Bee Wilson sums up how sweet foods and desserts can be used in our society to get children to do our bidding, stemming from a place of love: "Try a Brussels sprout and you can have dessert," "Practice piano and you have earned a chocolate bar," "You only get dessert if you've eaten everything on your plate." Candy is given out at schools as a reward for doing things like sweeping the classroom floor or listening well to instructions. Of course we want children to eat and try new foods, or do their best at school—so why not bribe them? It works in the moment most of the time—it's for their greater good and it is only sugar, right? A meta-analytic review of 128 studies examining the effects of extrinsic awards on intrinsic motivation revealed that all forms of rewards (food included) undermined free choice and intrinsic motivation (Deci, Koestner, and Ryan 1999). Children were much more likely to continue with an activity, or try hard and eat an unusual vegetable, if it had been initiated by their own free will. Self-motivation cannot be bought or bribed; it comes from deep within a child. Lao Tzu's quote applies here, "To vanquish others requires force, to vanquish self requires strength" (Tzu 2018). Parents and caregivers of children can succumb to the quick and easy power of sugar to exert control, or they can step back, master their own reactions and actions, and allow this intrinsic motivation to flourish without interference.

An excess of sweet treats in the diet also weakens Spleen *Qi* and creates conditions for dampness and phlegm in a child's body.

A US study found that 50 percent of children were exceeding the regular daily limit for sugar in their diet (Herrick *et al.* 2019). Experts and the WHO suggest that children should not exceed 25 grams (6 teaspoons) of sugar per day, and that children under two should have no added sugars in their diet. The main sources of these added sugars in the US study for infants were in yoghurt, baby snacks and sweets, and sweet bakery products, and for toddlers, the top sources were fruit drinks, sweet baked products, sugar, and candy. A cross-sectional survey of yoghurt sold in major UK supermarkets found that they varied widely in sugar content, and that only 2 percent of the children's brands were low enough in sugar to earn a green label, which indicates the healthier choice (Moore, Horti, and Fielding 2018).

Yang Sheng: *Yang Sheng*, which translates to "Nurturing Life," gives direction through its set of principles devoted to protecting the prenatal *Qi* and ways of nurturing the postnatal *Qi* through body, mind, and Spirit for harmony and health. Sun Simiao (581–682 CE) was dedicated to the art of *Yang Sheng*. *Yang Sheng* principles revolve around how we can all individually live our lives for longevity and to keep our bodies and spirit complete. *Yang Sheng* in relation to children's diets encompasses the parts found in this chapter, including adapting to the seasonal transitions, balancing, and including all five flavors and aiming to eat nutritious and nourishing foods. To nourish life also means to mainly choose from foods that are whole, unprocessed, and chemical-free. Where our food comes from matters—the life force of a freshly picked local food over one that has traveled hundreds of miles is obvious. Most farm animals raised today have not experienced a *Yang Sheng* way of life—they are raised in factory farms, crammed into cages, given antibiotics and hormones, or genetically manipulated to grow larger or to produce more eggs or milk than they normally would, and they don't have a chance to go outside, root around in the soil, or feel the sun on their bodies. Is it possible that we can eat this meat without transferring any of the suffering or fear they might have experienced into our spirit (*Shen*)? This remains an unanswered question, for now. Michael Pollan states,

> As long as one egg looks pretty much like another, all the chickens like chickens, and beef like beef, the substitution of quantity for quality will go

unnoticed by most consumers, but it is becoming increasingly apparent to anyone with an electron microscope or a mass spectrometer that, truly, this is not the same food. (2007, p.269)

CHAPTER 11

Recipes

Food is able to expel evil and stabilize the viscera and bowels, and to please the spirit and clear the will, thereby protecting blood and qi. If you are able to use food to balance out chronic disorders, release emotions, and chase away disease, you can call yourself an outstanding craftsperson. This is the special method of lengthening the years, and "eating for old age" and the utmost art of nurturing life...

Sun Simiao, *Bei Ji Qian Jin Yao Fang* (*Essential Prescriptions Worth a Thousand in Gold for Every Emergency*), translated by Sabine Wilms (2010)

There are so many resources for recipes these days. Bookstore shelves have cookbooks for every type of diet, cooking style, and how to make anything your heart desires; they are filled with mouth-watering imagery, tantalizing descriptions, and exotic ingredients. Online cooking blogs are ready to send you daily recipes with the insertion of your email address. Cooking shows and cooking challenges abound for adults as well as for children. Yet somehow, the practice of home cooking has been on the decline in the last few decades and is now rarely taught in school. The shift towards ready-to-eat food comes at a price to our health: "ready-to-eat meals have been linked to obesity and negative impacts on cognitive outcomes, particularly amongst children" (Crossley *et al.* 2018). Research has shown the importance of learning cooking skills at a young age before adolescence as it improves skill retention, confidence, cooking practices, cooking attitude, and diet quality in adulthood (Lavelle *et al.* 2016), which "may result in long-term benefits for nutritional well-being" (Utter *et al.* 2018). Eating home-cooked meals more frequently has been associated with better diet quality and lower adiposity (Mills *et al.* 2017). It is understandable that not everyone enjoys cooking, but hopefully, with the awareness of its links to better health outcomes, there might be a more concentrated effort to find ways to make it work; slow cookers, pressure cookers, and Instant Pots are all amazing kitchen aides for a busy family.

An emphasis on home cooking shows and cooking know-how is wonderful to see, and my hope is for this trend to continue to grow and spark a return to using less processed, pre-made ingredients in cooking. This will enable people to have a connection with what they are eating, and for children to be present in the kitchen, learning these culinary skills along the way.

Late spring, summer, autumn, winter, and the Spleen and Earth element

Many sources cite the Spleen and Earth to be associated with late summer, this being the time of year to nourish the Spleen. But why cut the summer short? It is a conundrum when trying to fit the five organs into four seasons. When looking at the Five Element phasic cycle it would make sense that Earth follows Fire, but when considering that Earth can also be looked at as the center, as the core of that which feeds our being, and thus all the organs, we can be content to realize that Earth, our root of digestion, needs continual replenishment all year long. Giovanni Maciocia writes, "what the Lei Jing says about the energy of the Spleen influencing the end of every season is more convincing. The Earth provides nourishment, and it makes sense that the Spleen should influence the end of every season" (1982, p.46). The last 18 days, then, of each season can be considered the Earth phase. With children, we can take it a step further and consider their first 18 years as their Earth phase—a continual focus on nourishing their Spleen and Stomach organs and postnatal *Qi*.

Considerations regarding food choices
Pesticides
The topic of pesticide use in our food system is a vast one, with conflicting information as to its safety. Governments assure us that all pesticide residues on foods are safe and that, to date, there is no health risk from eating conventionally grown produce because of pesticide residue (Government of Canada 2020). Glyphosate, the most widely used herbicide, was listed as a known carcinogen by the WHO in 2015. Glyphosate has also been shown to disrupt the gut microbiome in rat pups at the same dosages considered safe (Mao *et al.* 2018). And another study done with mice exposed to sub-

chronic and chronic amounts of glyphosate also found disruption in the gut microbiome that caused anxiety and depression-like behaviors (Aitbali *et al.* 2018). It is also becoming clearer that glyphosate is an endocrine disruptor that can alter female fertility (Ingaramo *et al.* 2020). Other research has shown that even low levels of pesticide exposure can affect young children's neurological and behavioral development (Liu and Schelar 2012). The European Union (EU) has moved forward with a strategy to reduce the use and risk of chemical and hazardous pesticides by 50 percent by 2030 (European Commission 2020). If they thought pesticides were 100 percent safe, they would not be trying to reduce their use. The good news is that after six days of eating organic produce, glyphosate was reduced by 70 percent in both children's and adults' bodies (Fagan *et al.* 2020; Hyland *et al.* 2020).

Organic produce can be an expensive endeavor, but there are ways to make it sustainable:

- Buying from local farmers markets; they may not be "certified" organic but are oftentimes unsprayed.
- Finding out which produce has higher amounts of pesticide use and buying only those organically grown (the Environmental Working Group (EWG) releases its tested "dirty dozen" online each year[1]).
- Frozen organic produce harvested at its peak can often be more affordable.

A group called the Detox Project[2] is testing and certifying foods that are glyphosate-free and working with governments to come up with solutions to chemical herbicides.

Food additives

Artificial flavor and food colorings: from nonedible food sources such as petroleum. Some examples are Red # 40, Yellow # 5, and Orange B. These have been shown to increase hyperactivity in children (Schab and Trinh 2004).

Natural flavor: from a natural source (plant or animal) to create specific flavors—the fourth most common ingredient on food labels (Andrews n.d.). Companies are not required to list what sources were used to derive the end product. Food manufacturers are increasingly using this manufactured

---

1   See www.ewg.org/
2   https://detoxproject.org/

ingredient to substitute the real item in processed foods. For example, natural blueberry flavor allows for no or very few blueberries in the product.

Carrageenan: extracted from seaweed and commonly used to thicken products such as sour cream, puddings, non-dairy milks, yoghurt, ice cream, cream, and infant formulas. This is a controversial ingredient that has been shown in animal studies to induce intestinal ulcers and human irritable bowel features (Martino, van Limbergen, and Cahill 2017; Watt and Marcus 1973). According to the WHO, however, it is considered a "safe" additive. If children present with chronic bowel issues, it is recommended eliminating this food additive for one month to assess any negative effect it may be having.

Bisphenols and bisphenol-free

Bisphenols are a group of chemicals used to manufacture plastics and epoxy resins. Bisphenol-A (BPA) is commonly used to make:

- Plastic, reusable water bottles.
- Plastic food storage containers.
- Older baby bottles and sippy cups (though its use in baby bottles is now banned).
- Lining inside canned food products.
- Coating on sales receipts.

Due to the endocrine-disrupting nature of BPA (a known xenoestrogen, in that it processes estrogenic and anti-androgenic properties), many products are now labeled as BPA-free. There have been many alternatives for BPA in products, such as, BPS, BPF, and BPAF; they all begin with BP because they share the same basic chemical structure as bisphenol. Some studies have shown these alternatives still have endocrine-disrupting effects (Eladak *et al.* 2015; Mao *et al.* 2020; Rochester and Bolden 2015). BPA and its substitutes cross through the placenta to the fetus in pregnant women in high concentrations. No one really understands the effects this may have on brain and reproductive development (Pan *et al.* 2020).

The best ways to reduce BPA and BPA-free exposure in babies and children are as follows:

- Use glass or stainless containers for food storage and lunches and snacks.
- Use glass or stainless water bottles.

- Look for canned food that is *not* lined with BPA—many companies have switched to lining their cans with acrylic and polyester forms of plastic. The best solution, however, is to reduce canned food consumption. Beans can be cooked in a pressure cooker and tomato sauce and tomatoes bought in glass jars or frozen.

The recipes

In this chapter there are basic recipe ideas for nourishing breakfast, lunch, dinner, and snacks that are moderately easy to create and serve to cater to the tastes of a young child's often selective palette. The recipes include the Chinese dietary principles, and the icons denote the recipes' seasonal attunement. Bon appétit!

❄️ Winter   ☀️ Summer

🌱 Spring   🍃 Autumn

Breakfast

BIRCHER MÜESLI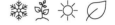
Gluten-free, vegetarian, vegan

A traditional Swiss breakfast that is almost perfect. Because the breakfast soaks overnight, it is ready to eat in the morning, but since it is usually served cold, it needs to be slightly tweaked. Yoghurt is moistening and nourishes *Yin*. Millet nourishes *Qi* and Kidney *Yin*. Quinoa nourishes Spleen *Qi* and tonifies Kidney *Yang*. Rye dries dampness and nourishes *Qi*. Oats nourish Spleen and Stomach and tonify *Qi* and Blood.

Ingredients
- 3 cups of unsweetened yoghurt
- 1 apple
- 1 pear
- ¾ cup of millet flakes, quinoa flakes, rye flakes, rolled oats or a combination
- ¼ cup of raisins, or chopped dried fruit of choice
- 2 cups of seasonal fruit (omit in the winter)
- ½ cup of chopped nuts or seeds

- 1 tsp cinnamon
- Optional: can add a little sweetener if required (honey, maple syrup)

Method

1. Core and grate the apple and pear immediately into the yoghurt to prevent browning.
2. Mix in the grain flakes, the dried fruit, the seasonal fruit (if using) and the nuts or seeds. Mix in the cinnamon.
3. Stir to combine, and refrigerate overnight.
4. In the morning heat on the stove and serve immediately.

BUTTERMILK PANCAKES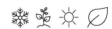

Nut-free, vegetarian, vegan

This is a weekend specialty that can be healthful. Making the batter from scratch makes it even more so. Spelt flour is nourishing to Spleen *Qi*. Warming spices can be used to stimulate digestion and for flavoring, and in the summer seasonal berries and fruit can be used as a topping.

Ingredients

- 1 cup of buttermilk (or add 1 tbsp lemon juice or apple cider vinegar to 1 cup of milk, dairy or non-dairy, and let it sit for 10 minutes)
- 1 cup of spelt flour
- 1½ tsp baking powder
- ½ tsp baking soda
- 1½ tsp spices (e.g. ¾ tsp cinnamon, ¼ tsp nutmeg, ¼ tsp ginger, ¼ tsp cardamom blended or pumpkin pie spice blend)
- ¼ tsp salt
- 1 tsp olive oil
- 1 egg (can be omitted)
- Butter or oil
- Seasonal fruit
- Maple syrup, to sweeten

Method

1. Mix the dry ingredients in a bowl with a whisk.
2. Beat the egg and add to the milk, along with the olive oil.
3. Whisk the egg and milk into the dry ingredients, to form a batter. Let batter rest at room temperature for 5 to 30 minutes.

4. Drop a spoonful of batter onto a griddle or a lightly buttered or oiled pan set to medium or medium low. The mix will make about 8–10 small pancakes.

5. Chop the fruit and top the pancake with fruit and maple syrup.

MILLET MUESLI[3]

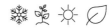

Gluten-free, vegetarian, vegan

When it comes to the eating habits of children, the first years of life are formative. Eating skills develop from sucking and swallowing, to introducing solid food, to eating with the hands, and finally to actively participating in meals at the table (family or daycare). Children are guided by the example of adults, and develop preferences, which is why they should be introduced at an early stage to a balanced and healthy diet as well as to the joy and habit of communal times at the table.

From a TCM point of view, the most important foods for children's growth are those that support the Middle Burner. Therefore, neutral to slightly warming foods with sweet flavors are ideal for children, while energetically cool and cold foods should be avoided. In general, warm foods are easier to digest and cold or raw foods should be avoided, especially for young children.

Colorful foods should also be emphasized; not only do children like them but colors also support the organ functions. The Spleen, for example, is supported by yellow, so you will want to add yellow fruits, vegetables, or nuts and seeds to meals as often as possible.

Muesli strengthens and warms the Middle Burner and it protects against too much moisture, especially in autumn and winter. This breakfast tonifies Spleen-pancreas energy and Stomach *Qi* deliciously all year long and strengthens Kidney *Yang*. Cinnamon moves *Qi* and *Xue* and tonifies Kidney *Yang*; raisins are warming, have a strong effect on the Kidneys and Liver, and tonify *Qi* and blood.

Ingredients

- ½ cup of millet
- 2¼–2½ cups of water
- Toppings:

---

3   This recipe was generously submitted from Angelika-Marie Findgott, author of *Five Elements in the Kitchen: Recipes from My Friends in Chinese Medicine.*

- 3 tbsp raisins
- 1 tbsp cinnamon
- Optional toppings and supplements (depending on the season and preferences): fresh, stewed, or dried fruit (pears, bananas, apples, plums, apricots...), honey, maple syrup, almonds, sunflower seeds, pumpkin seeds, sesame seeds, walnuts.

Method

1. Rinse the millet under cold running water.
2. Add the water to a saucepan, cover and bring to the boil.
3. Add the millet, and bring to a second boil.
4. Let the millet simmer for 20–30 minutes, until all the water is absorbed. It should be a little moist and not too grainy. The more water used, the softer the millet.
5. While the millet is boiling, set up the table with small dishes of the toppings and supplements.
6. Portion out the millet to individual bowls, and top as you like best.

NUT-ELLA

Gluten-free (use maple syrup), vegetarian, vegan (use nut milk)

This homemade version is nothing like the store-bought kind. With the amount of sugar in the store-bought version, spreading it on toast is akin to slathering icing on children's breakfasts in the mornings. It does take a little time to make at home, but many hands make light work, and this recipe is one children can easily help with, even the littler hands. Hazelnuts are nourishing to the Spleen and Stomach and have a neutral thermal nature. They impart a harmonizing effect on the digestive system and are indicated when there is a lack of appetite. Walnut oil is warming and nourishes Kidney *Yang*. If there are any signs of hyperactivity, substitute carob powder for the cocoa powder. Cocoa is stimulating and strengthening, while carob has a warming thermal nature. This is a breakfast staple in our house through the colder months of the year.

Ingredients

- 2 cups of hazelnuts
- 2 tbsp walnut oil (can also use olive or coconut oil)
- 2 tbsp barley malt (can also use maple syrup)

- ½ cup of unsweetened cocoa powder (can also use carob powder)
- 1 cup of milk

Method

1. Preheat the oven to 350°F.
2. Spread the hazelnuts on a rimmed baking sheet, and roast for 8 minutes. Remove from the oven and leave to cool. This is where all the hands come in handy—it's time to remove as much loose skin as possible from the hazelnuts. You can use a towel to roll them in to loosen the skins. Not all of it will come off, and that's okay.
3. Grind the hazelnuts in a blender until they form a paste.
4. Add the rest of the ingredients and continue to process until the mixture is as smooth as possible. You may need to add a little more milk depending on the consistency.
5. This will store refrigerated in an airtight container for several weeks (if it lasts that long!).
6. Enjoy spread over toast, pancakes, or just a spoonful for a blast of protein.

SCRAMBLED TOFU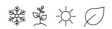

Gluten-free, nut-free, vegetarian, vegan

Tofu is cooling, benefits the Lungs and Large Intestine and is a complete protein. If children are eating tofu regularly, it is important to find out how it's being cooked, as it quite cooling in nature. The addition of warming spices will help to warm it up. Turmeric, which is warming, is used in this recipe to add the yellow coloring, but if children don't like it, then paprika, which is also warming, can be used instead. Nutritional yeast stimulates digestion, is high in fiber and rich in vitamin B12.

Ingredients

- 1 tbsp olive oil or butter
- 1¾ cup of firm or extra-firm tofu
- 2 tbsp nutritional yeast
- ¼ tsp turmeric (or paprika)
- 2 tbsp unsweetened milk
- ½ tsp salt
- Seasonal vegetables (such as red or yellow peppers, zucchini (also known as courgettes), broccoli, dark leafy greens)

Method

1. Heat the oil or butter in saucepan over a medium heat.
2. Add seasonal vegetables at the start of cooking with the oil or butter (before the tofu is added).
3. Crumble the tofu with your hands or mash with a fork and add to the saucepan. Cook, stirring frequently, until water from the tofu has reduced—about 3–4 minutes.
4. Add the remaining ingredients and continue to cook for another 5 minutes, stirring constantly to avoid burning.
5. Pour the milk into the saucepan and stir to mix in.
6. This can be served with toast.

SIMPLE GRANOLA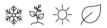

Gluten-free (use gluten-free oats), vegetarian, vegan

This is simple to make in large batches and could also be enjoyed as a snack. Yoghurt can be added on top (let it sit for 15 minutes to allow the yoghurt to "warm up," or add a little boiling hot water) along with seasonal fruit. If milk is used, first warm the milk up on the stove before adding. Granola can also be used to add spices therapeutically—for instance, ¼ tsp ground cloves, ¼ tsp nutmeg, ½ tsp cardamom along with the cinnamon. Oats are neutral in temperature and nourish the Spleen, strengthen the nerves and tonify *Qi*. Coconut is cooling and clears heat. Raisins are warming, nourish the *Qi* and the Blood, and benefit the Liver and Kidneys. Cinnamon warms the *Yang*.

Ingredients

- 4 cups of rolled oats
- 1 cup of mixed nuts
- ½ cup of olive oil
- ½ cup of maple syrup
- ⅓ cup of coconut flakes
- 1 tsp salt
- 1 cup of seeds
- ⅔ cup of raisins
- 1 tsp cinnamon

Method

1. Preheat the oven to 350°F.
2. Mix the oats, nuts, olive oil, maple syrup, coconut flakes, and salt. Spread over a baking sheet.
3. Bake for 20–25 minutes until golden brown, stirring halfway through.
4. Add the seeds, raisins, and cinnamon.
5. This stores in an airtight container for up to two weeks.

SUMMER MUNG BEAN BREAKFAST SOUP

Gluten-free, nut-free, vegetarian, vegan

Mung beans are the quintessential summer cooling remedy. As soon as the sun starts to beat down daily, this breakfast will help to prevent summer heat issues. Children are particularly sensitive to heat. Mung beans are cooling, detoxifying, and benefit the Liver and Gallbladder. They increase *Yin* fluids in the body but reduce damp-heat. Coconut milk nourishes *Qi*, builds stamina, nourishes blood, *Yin*, and *Jing*, and promotes proper growth and development.

Ingredients

- 1 cup of of mung beans (soaked overnight)
- 5 cups of water
- 1 can of organic coconut milk
- Honey, to taste
- Can top with fresh seasonal berries

Method

1. Drain the beans and place in a saucepan with the water. Bring to a boil.
2. Reduce the heat and simmer for 30 minutes.
3. Turn off the heat, add the coconut milk and let sit for an additional 10 minutes.
4. Add honey, if necessary, and serve with toppings of choice.

School lunch and snack ideas

APPLE MUFFINS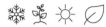
Nut-free, vegetarian, vegan

Apples are sweet and sour, benefit the Lungs, help to produce fluids for the body, and stimulate appetite.

Ingredients
- 1¾ cup of flour (spelt, whole wheat, or other)
- 1 cup of grated apple
- 1 cup of diced apple
- ½ cup of applesauce
- ½ cup of maple syrup
- ⅓ cup of oil
- 2 eggs (or 2 tbsp ground flax seeds mixed with 6 tbsp water)
- ½ cup of Greek yoghurt (or coconut yoghurt)
- ½ tsp salt
- 1½ tsp baking powder
- ½ tsp baking soda
- 1 tsp cinnamon
- 1 tsp vanilla

Method
1. Preheat the oven to 425°F.
2. Mix the flour, salt, baking powder, baking soda and cinnamon together.
3. Beat the eggs (or mixed flax seeds and water), add in the maple syrup, applesauce, oil, vanilla, and yoghurt.
4. Add the wet ingredients to the dry ingredients and incorporate.
5. Fold in the grated and diced apple.
6. Bake for 13–16 minutes. This recipe makes 12 muffins.

BLACK BEAN BROWNIES
Gluten-free, nut-free

These brownies are made without flour! Black beans are used in place of flour and are the main ingredient; they nourish Kidney *Yin*, build Blood, and have a warming thermal nature. Black beans are high in fiber and contain resistant starches that act as prebiotics to help feed the beneficial bacteria in the gut. Eggs are neutral in thermal nature, tonify Blood and *Yin*, and are indicated for dryness in the upper body (throat and Lungs) These brownies can also be made into muffins by spooning the batter into a lined muffin tin and reducing the baking time by 5 minutes to 20 minutes.

Ingredients
- 1¾ cup of cooked black beans
- 3 large eggs
- ⅔ cup of maple syrup (or use 15 pitted dates, chopped)
- 3 tbsp walnut or olive oil
- ¼ cup of cocoa
- 1 tsp vanilla
- ½ tsp baking powder
- ¼ tsp salt

Method
1. Preheat the oven to 350°F.
2. Blend all the ingredients in a food processor.
3. Line a 9 x 9 inch baking pan with parchment paper hanging over the sides.
4. Pour the mixture into the pan.
5. Bake for 25 minutes until a toothpick inserted in the center comes out clean.

BLISS SEED BALLS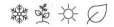
Gluten-free, nut-free, vegetarian, vegan

All the seeds in these balls are wonderfully nourishing for children's *Yin*. Grounding and healthy, this snack will help children focus. Hemp seeds are a traditional TCM medicine for constipation. They are sweet in flavor and neutral in thermal nature. Sunflowers nourish Spleen *Qi*, chia seeds nourish Kidney *Yin*, sesame seeds nourish blood and *Yin*. Dates are sweet and nourish Spleen *Qi* and blood. Coconut is warming, sweet, and tonifies the Heart.

Ingredients
- 1 cup of pitted dates
- ½ cup of raisins

- ¼ cup of sunflower seeds
- 2 tbsp hemp seeds
- 2 tbsp chia seeds
- 2 tbsp cocoa or carob powder
- 1 tbsp coconut oil
- Enough shredded coconut to roll bars in (can also roll balls in cocoa or carob to coat)

Method

1. Pour hot water over the dates and let sit for 10 minutes. Drain well.
2. Put all the seeds into a food processor and blend.
3. Add the dates, raisins, cocoa or carob, coconut oil and process until well blended.
4. Form into balls, and then roll in shredded coconut to coat.

CRACKERS (HOMEMADE)[4]

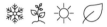

Gluten free, nut-free, vegetarian, vegan

It's hard to find nutritious crackers and when I do the price tag is usually shocking! These crackers have none of the extras of the highly processed versions. Brown rice nourishes Spleen *Qi* and quinoa is great for children as it strongly nourishes Spleen *Qi* and Kidney *Yang*.

Ingredients

- 2 cups of cooked brown rice
- 2 cups of cooked quinoa
- ⅔ cup of sunflower seeds
- ½ cup of flax seeds
- 2 tbsp tamari
- 3 tbsp olive oil
- 1 tsp salt

Method

1. Soak the flax seeds for 20 minutes in ½ cup of water.
2. Preheat the oven to 350°F.
3. Toast the sesame seeds in a skillet until lightly browned.
4. Place the cooled brown rice, quinoa, soaked flax seeds, tamari, salt,

---

4   Recipe from Sarah Britton, www.mynewroots.org/site/2012/05/happy-crackers-2/

and olive oil into a food processor and blend until a dough forms. If the mixture is dry, add a little water at a time.

5. Add the sesame seeds and pulse a few more times. The dough will be sticky. Take the dough out and place onto parchment paper. Taste and add more salt if required.

6. Put another piece of parchment on top and roll out until it's a very thin, even form. Remove the top parchment, and with a knife score the dough into desired shapes and sizes (great time for heart shapes!).

7. Carefully slide the parchment onto a baking sheet and bake in the oven for about 30 minutes—check after 25 minutes.

8. Remove from the oven and leave to cool.

9. Break along the score lines. If some crackers are still uncooked, place back in the oven for a little longer.

10. Store in an airtight container; keeps for one week.

CUCUMBER SALAD

Gluten free, nut-free, vegetarian, vegan

Children enjoy simplicity, and this salad delivers. Cucumber is cold, bitter, and clears heat—perfect to balance the Heart in the summer months. Rice wine vinegar is also bitter and helps to move Liver *Qi*. Children should only have a small amount of this salad to protect their Middle Burners.

Ingredients
- 3 English cucumbers, sliced thinly
- 2 tbsp rice wine vinegar
- 1 tbsp sesame seeds

Method
1. Place all the ingredients into a bowl. Toss to combine.

HUMMUS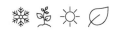

Gluten free, nut-free, vegetarian, vegan

Hummus is usually enjoyed by children, is protein-rich, and a great source of fiber. Chickpeas nourish both Spleen and Kidney *Qi* and are neutral in thermal nature. This is a wonderful dip to have on a regular basis. I reduce or eliminate the garlic in my version, as I find garlic to be a little too "heating" for children. In the summer, raw vegetables can be used to dip, and through the rest of the seasons, on crackers, rice cakes, spread on bread, or used in a wrap.

Ingredients
- 3 cups of chickpeas (2 x 15 oz cans)
- ¼ cup of olive oil
- ½ cup of tahini or ½ cup of sesame seeds
- 2 tbsp lime juice (can also use lemon juice)
- ½ clove garlic, crushed
- Pinch of paprika
- 1 tsp cumin
- ¼ tsp salt
- Cold water as needed to thin
- Alternatives: Can add chopped cilantro (coriander) or parsley as a topping

Method
1. Puree the chickpeas, tahini or sesame seeds, lime juice, garlic, salt, and spices in a food processor. Blend until smooth.
2. Add the olive oil and pulse a few more times until just combined.
3. Add a little bit of cold water if the consistency is too thick.

KALE SUNFLOWER CHIPS[5]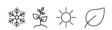
Gluten-free, nut-free, vegetarian, vegan

These are a cinch to make and easy for children to love. Kale is a powerhouse of nutrients—one cup gives you more than the recommended daily amount of vitamin C (helps cuts and wounds heal faster, and keeps the immune system strong), A (important for normal growth and vision), and K (blood-clotting function). Great for children as it nourishes Spleen *Qi* and benefits the Stomach. I pop these into a warm oven (just need to remember to turn it down) after cooking dinner, and they are ready as snacks for the next day.

Ingredients
- 1 large bunch of kale

---

5   Recipe generously submitted from Lindsey Youell, a friend and certified nutritional counsellor in Victoria, BC.

- ¼ cup of oil
- 2 tbsp nutritional yeast
- 1 tbsp lemon juice
- ¼ cup of sunflower seeds
- Salt to taste

Method

1. Preheat the oven to 350°F.
2. Tear the leaves off the kale and save the stems in the freezer for a future soup stock.
3. Rinse well and dry in a salad spinner and then pat dry with a lint free cloth or paper towel to remove as much moisture as possible.
4. In a blender, combine all the other ingredients.
5. In a big bowl, add the sauce to the kale and massage it in.
6. Spread the kale leaves apart on a rimmed baking sheet lined with parchment paper. Roast for 10 minutes. Flip halfway through for even cooking. Watch carefully as kale burns quickly in the oven.
7. These are best eaten within 24 hours as they lose their crispiness after that.
8. Store in an airtight container.

OAT AND CARDAMOM MUFFINS

Gluten-free, nut-free, vegetarian, vegan

Oats are nourishing to Spleen and Stomach *Qi*. Cardamom is warming and drying, goes to the Lungs, and resolves phlegm. Cardamom also stimulates digestion.

Ingredients

- 1½ cups of oat flour (can blend rolled oats in a food processor to make oat flour)
- ½ cup of milk (dairy or non-dairy)
- 1 tsp apple cider vinegar
- 1 tbsp ground cardamom
- 2 eggs (or mix 2 tbsp ground flax seeds with 6 tbsp water)
- ¼ cup of walnut or olive oil
- ¼ cup of applesauce
- ½ cup of raw cane sugar

- 1¼ tsp baking powder
- ½ tsp baking soda
- ½ tsp salt
- Can top with pumpkin seeds or chocolate chips

Method

1. Preheat the oven to 350°F.
2. Add the vinegar to the milk and let sit for 10 minutes.
3. Mix the dry ingredients together.
4. In a separate bowl, whisk or beat the eggs, and add the sugar until blended.
5. Add the oil and applesauce and continue to beat.
6. With the mixer on low or continuing to hand whisk, add half the flour mixture to the wet ingredients, then add half the milk and vinegar until combined, then add the rest of the flour and milk and vinegar, and beat until combined to make a batter.
7. Spoon the batter into a lined muffin tin. Top with pumpkin seeds or chocolate chips. This recipe makes 12 muffins.
8. Bake for about 20–25 minutes.

OATMEAL AND SESAME SEED CHOCOLATE CHIP COOKIES

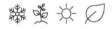

Nut-free, vegetarian

Every child needs a chocolate chip in their life! These are a healthier version of the traditional cookie. Oats are warming and nourish Spleen and Stomach *Qi* and benefit the nerves. Sesame seeds nourish the *Yin* of all the organs, and particularly benefit the Liver and Kidneys.

Ingredients

- 1 cup of oats
- ¾ cup of flour (whole wheat, spelt, or other)
- ¼ cup of tahini
- ¼ cup of maple syrup
- 2 tbsp milk (dairy or non-dairy)
- ¼ cup of sesame seeds
- ½ cup of chocolate chips
- 1 egg (or mix 1 tbsp ground flax seed with 3 tbsp water)

- 1 tsp baking powder
- 1 tsp vanilla
- ¼ tsp salt

Method
1. Preheat the oven to 350°F.
2. Mix all the ingredients together in a bowl.
3. After mixing, let the dough sit for 10 minutes in the fridge.
4. Drop by the spoonful onto a baking sheet lined with parchment paper. Bake for 12–15 minutes.

PEAR JUICE[6]

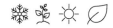

Gluten-free, nut-free, vegetarian, vegan

Deirdre Courtney uses pears when there are Lung issues in children. Pears benefit the Lungs, clear heat, and transform phlegm. Apples also benefit the Lungs. Celery clears heat.

Ingredients
- 2 organic pears
- Juice of one lime
- Half to 1 stick of celery, depending if there is heat or not
- Small piece of ginger
- Half an apple
- Small amount of water to thin

Method
1. Juice all the ingredients. Add water to thin.

---

6   Recipe generously submitted from Deirdre Courtney, author of *Nourishing Life the Yang Sheng Way* and a practitioner of Chinese Medicine, Acupuncture, Herbalism, Nutrition and Tui na, and a specialist in Face Reading, Facial Diagnosis, Rejuvenation, and *Yang Sheng*.

PEAR SMOOTHY[7]

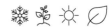

Gluten-free, nut-free, vegetarian

Deirdre Courtney uses pears and almonds for chronic Lung issues with children.

Ingredients

- 1 organic pear, cored, skin left on
- 6–10 almonds (substitute with sunflower, pumpkin, or hemp seeds or 1 tsp raw almond butter)
- ½ cup of almond milk (or hemp milk), or ¼ avocado mixed with some water
- Honey to taste, local (if possible) and only if the child is old enough
- Pinch of turmeric (if possible, but a lot of young children don't like it)
- Additions: Blueberries are good for all organs; apricots are good for Lungs; papaya is good for digestion

Method

1. Blend all the ingredients in a food processor.

POPCORN (HOMEMADE)

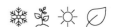

Gluten-free, nut-free, vegetarian, vegan

This popcorn is made on the stove, eliminating the need for bagged popcorn, most of which is lined with chemicals that are probably not conducive to health. Popcorn is high in fiber and can be topped with nutritional yeast for added vitamins. Popcorn is not a traditional TCM food, but due to its ease for snacking and Western popularity I have included it. I am sure popcorn benefits digestion due to its ability to feed the microbiome.

Ingredients

- ½ cup of popcorn kernels
- 2 tbsp olive or coconut oil

---

7   Recipe generously submitted from Deirdre Courtney, author of *Nourishing Life the Yang Sheng Way* and a practitioner of Chinese Medicine, Acupuncture, Herbalism, Nutrition and Tui na, and a specialist in Face Reading, Facial Diagnosis, Rejuvenation, and *Yang Sheng*.

Method

1. Heat the oil over a medium heat in a deep saucepan that has a lid.
2. Drop two popcorn kernels into the saucepan to begin with, to know when the oil is hot enough (look for when they pop out). Add the rest of the popcorn kernels and place the lid partway on (to allow steam to escape); shake the pan vigorously to keep the kernels moving.
3. When the kernels start to pop, remove briefly from the heat so as not to burn, then place the pan back on and off until all the kernels have popped.
4. Sprinkle nutritional yeast over before serving.
5. If using coconut oil you can sprinkle with cinnamon.

PUFFED AMARANTH AND SEED BAR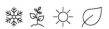

Gluten-free, nut-free, vegetarian

Amaranth has a high nutritional value, is a high source of protein, is high in iron and magnesium, has great fiber, and is gluten-free. Amaranth grain is highly nutritious and a great building block for children; it is high in Lysine that supports healthy growth and development. Amaranth benefits the Lungs and strengthens *Qi*. Pumpkin seeds are warming, moisten the Intestines, and are a known remedy for eliminating intestinal parasites. Sesame seeds nourish Blood and *Yin*. These are a great alternative to store-bought bars that can be low in nutrition.

Ingredients

- 6 cups of puffed amaranth (about 1¼ cups of dried amaranth)
- 1¼ cups of raw cane sugar
- ¼ cup of honey
- ½ cup of water
- ½ cup of pumpkin seeds (can toast if preferred)
- ½ cup of sesame seeds, black or white (can toast if preferred)
- 1 tbsp lime juice

Method

1. Puffed amaranth can either be bought or made at home. It pops quickly but it does take a little practice to get it right. Heat a heavy-bottomed, high-sided saucepan on medium-high heat. The pan must be sizzling hot before adding the amaranth. Have a lid nearby ready to use.

2. Add 1–2 tsp of amaranth at a time, shaking the pan constantly. Place the lid partly over the top of the pan while continuing to shake (using one hand for each). The amaranth should pop and turn a whitish colour, and once popping has started it should take about 10–15 seconds for all the grains to pop. Empty the puffed amaranth into a bowl and continue with another 1–2 tsp of amaranth until all is popped.
3. Line a 9 x 9 inch baking pan with parchment paper.
4. Blend the puffed amaranth, pumpkin and sesame seeds and salt in a large bowl.
5. Mix the sugar, honey, and water in a saucepan and heat over medium-high heat until boiling.
6. Remove from the heat, stir in the lime juice and while still liquid, pour over the puffed amaranth blend. Mix in well.
7. Transfer to the baking pan and press down using a spatula.
8. Place in the freezer for 30 minutes to set, then cut into squares.

ROASTED CHICKPEAS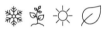

Gluten-free, nut-free, vegetarian, vegan

Easy to pack in lunches, eat as a snack, add to wraps, eat as a side dish—they are delightfully crispy and wonderfully nourishing. Chickpeas have more iron than other legumes, are beneficial for the gut flora, and nourish the Spleen and Stomach. They are sweet and neutral in thermal nature.

Ingredients
- 3 cups of cooked chickpeas (2 x 15 oz cans)
- 2 tbsp olive oil
- ½ tsp salt
- 4 tsp dried spice of choice, depending on season

Method
1. Preheat the oven to 400°F.
2. Pat the chickpeas dry and remove any loose skin.
3. Lay the chickpeas flat on a parchment-lined baking tray. Drizzle with olive oil and salt to evenly coat.
4. Roast for 20–30 minutes until golden brown and slightly darker in places—soft on the inside, crispy on the outside; *Yin, Yang* balance.

SPINACH AND CHIVE MUFFINS

Nut-free, vegetarian

Spinach nourishes the blood and *Yin* and clears heat. These muffins pack well for lunches and offer a nutritious snack. Chives move blood and warm the Stomach.

Ingredients
- 1 tbsp olive oil
- 4 cups of spinach
- 3 chive stalks
- 1⅓ cups of flour (spelt, whole wheat, or other)
- 2 tsp baking powder
- 3 heaped tbsp Parmesan cheese
- 1 egg (or mix 1 tbsp ground flax seeds with 3 tbsp water)
- ⅔ cup of milk (dairy or non-dairy)
- ¼ cup of butter, ghee, or olive oil
- 3 heaped tbsp cottage cheese
- ½ tsp salt
- A little black pepper

Method
1. Preheat the oven to 350°F.
2. Line a muffin pan with 8 liners.
3. Heat the oil in pan and add the spinach to wilt. Cook for a few minutes.
4. Finely chop the chives.
5. Mix the flour, baking powder, Parmesan cheese, salt, and pepper.
6. In a separate bowl whisk the milk and melted butter, ghee, or olive oil, and add the egg (or ground flax seeds and water).
7. Mix with the dry ingredients.
8. Fold in the spinach, chives, and cottage cheese.
9. Fill the liners two-thirds full. Bake for 30 minutes.

SWEET POTATO TOAST

Gluten-free, nut-free, vegetarian

A healthy alternative to bread, sweet potatoes are deeply nourishing to the Spleen and Stomach. This "toast" can be topped with an avocado and an egg, or just some cheese with a sprinkle of paprika. Avocados are cooling and moistening and eggs are warming and nourish *Qi* and Blood. Paprika promotes and warms the digestion. You can roast extra sweet potato—it keeps in the fridge for a couple of days and can be quickly reheated to use for a few breakfasts (you can even pop them into the toaster for a quicker reheat).

Ingredients
- 1 large sweet potato or yam
- 1 tbsp olive or coconut oil
- 1 avocado
- 4 eggs
- Salt, pepper, pinch of paprika

Method
1. Preheat the oven to 400°F.
2. Cut the potatoes in ½ inch slices along the long part. There should be about 4 slices with 2 little ends cut off.
3. Brush the potatoes with oil. Roast for about 15 minutes, flipping over halfway through cooking.
4. Cook the eggs as preferred.
5. Smash the avocado and add a pinch of salt, pepper, and paprika.
6. Once cooked, top the sweet potatoes with avocado, egg, or a little cheese and paprika.

STEWED APPLE AND PEAR[8]

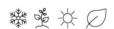

Gluten-free, nut-free, vegetarian, vegan

Deirdre Courtney uses apples and pears when there are Lung issues in children as they both benefit the Lungs. This recipe is better for younger children but can also be a snack for older ones.

Ingredients
- 2 organic apples
- 2 organic pears
- 2 tbsp water

---

8   Recipe generously submitted from Deirdre Courtney author of *Nourishing Life the Yang Sheng Way* and a practitioner of Chinese Medicine, Acupuncture, Herbalism, Nutrition and Tui na, and a specialist in Face Reading, Facial Diagnosis, Rejuvenation and *Yang Sheng*.

Method

1. Core the apples and pears.
2. Slice and place in a saucepan with the water.
3. Turn the heat to medium to low. Cook for about 20 minutes, stirring occasionally.
4. Leave to cool and then puree with a hand blender.

WINTER SQUASH LOAF (PUMPKIN, BUTTERNUT, OR KABOCHA)

Nut-free, vegetarian, vegan

Winter squash, in all their shades of green, orange, yellow, brown, gray, and white autumn colors, are beautiful to look at, store well through the winter, and are high on the list of foods that nourish the Spleen and Stomach *Qi*. They are naturally sweet and have a warming thermal nature; pumpkin, though, has a cooling thermal nature. Pureed squash is a wonderful first food for babies as it is so full of nutrition and easy to digest. Squash contain an abundance of carotenoids, which are potent antioxidants. One of them, beta-carotene, is the precursor to vitamin A, which helps with children's growth and development and is particularly important in supporting vision and regulating immunity.

Ingredients

- 1 cup of squash puree
- ⅓ cup of olive oil
- 1 large egg or two small eggs (or mix 1 tbsp ground flax seeds with 3 tbsp water)
- ½ cup of Greek yoghurt (or coconut yoghurt)
- ½ cup of honey or maple syrup
- 1 cup of flour (whole wheat, spelt)
- ½ cup of oat flour (add rolled oats to a food processor and blend until a fine flour has formed)
- 2 tsp pumpkin spice blend (1 tsp cinnamon, ½ tsp nutmeg, ¼ tsp ground ginger, ⅛ tsp ground cloves, all blended together)
- 1 tsp baking soda
- ¼ tsp salt
- ¼ cup of chocolate chips (or vegan chocolate chips)
- ¼ cup of chopped nuts (walnuts, pecans, or hazelnuts)

Method

1. Preheat the oven to 350°F.
2. Grease a 9 x 5 inch loaf pan with butter or oil and line with parchment paper.
3. Combine the squash puree, egg, oil, yoghurt, and honey or maple syrup in a bowl and use a hand mixer to beat together.
4. In a separate bowl, combine all the dry ingredients.
5. Mix the wet and dry ingredients together until just combined (over-mixing will create a dense loaf).
6. Pour into a loaf pan and bake for 45–60 minutes.

Home lunch and dinner ideas

ANELLINI PASTA WITH BROCCOLI AND HAM[9]

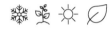

Nut-free

This is a nourishing recipe that Lillian Pearl Bridges makes for her grandchildren. Children love pasta and I have yet to meet a child who won't eat it! Broccoli is slightly bitter and cool, and cools the Liver and Blood. Ham (pork) supplements the *Yin* and blood. Parmesan cheese contains probiotics that are beneficial for the gut microbiome.

Ingredients

- 1 cup of Anellini pasta (or another small pasta shape)
- 1 cup of cooked broccoli, chopped
- 1 cup of ham, chopped
- ½ tsp garlic, crushed
- 6 tbsp salted butter
- Optional: Parmesan cheese for serving

Method

1. Boil the Anellini pasta in a saucepan of salted boiling water until done (according to the package directions) and then drain.
2. In the meantime, in a frying pan, melt the butter and add the garlic.
3. Cook until you can smell the garlic fragrance well.

---

9   Recipe generously submitted from Lillian Pearl Bridges, author of *Face Reading in Chinese Medicine*.

4. Add the ham and broccoli and cook until hot.
5. Add the drained pasta when done and stir to combine, reheating if necessary.
6. Serve with Parmesan cheese.

CABBAGE, THE GERMAN WAY (ROTKRAUT) ❄ ⚘ ☼ ⬭
Gluten-free, nut-free, vegetarian, vegan

Cabbage has a sweet and pungent flavor, improves digestion, is high in vitamin C, and it contains insoluble fiber that helps to support the gut bacteria. Cabbage is moistening to the Intestines and can be used for constipation. Lemon juice is sour and benefits the Liver. Apple cider vinegar is also sour and benefits the Liver.

Ingredients
− 1 head of red cabbage
− 1 organic tart apple
− 3 tbsp olive oil (or butter)
− ½ cup of apple cider vinegar
− ½ cup of water
− ½ cup of honey
− ¼ tsp black pepper
− Pinch of ground cloves
− 3 juniper berries
− 1 bay leaf
− ½ tsp salt
− 1 tbsp lemon juice
− Flour (or gluten-free flour)

Method
1. Cut the cabbage in half. Cut out the tough, white center, then cut each half again. Very finely shred the four pieces of cabbage.
2. Cut and grate the apple.
3. Heat the oil or butter in a saucepan. Add the cabbage and sauté for 5 minutes.
4. Add the apple, vinegar, honey, pepper, cloves, juniper berries, bay leaf, salt, and water.
5. Cover and bring to a boil over a medium heat.

6. Reduce and simmer for 30–45 minutes, until the cabbage is tender. This can also be made in the pressure cooker with a 5-minute cooking time.
7. Stir in the lemon juice.
8. Just before serving, sprinkle a little flour over the cabbage to absorb the liquid. Use gluten-free flour if required.

CARROT SALAD

Gluten-free, nut-free, vegetarian, vegan

My daughter's school mate lived in France with her family for a year and attended school there. She was in kindergarten at the time and her mom would post photos and blog about their experience. I was in awe when I saw their school hot lunch menu; lunches were available daily if desired and the menu was diverse and could have been posted at a French bistro. The grated carrot salad caught my eye as such a wonderful way to serve raw carrots to children instead of serving them as carrot sticks. The chicken cordon bleu also caught my attention; what a wonderful way for these children to have a healthy hot lunch each school day! Carrots strengthen the Spleen and benefit the Lungs.

Ingredients
- 3½ cups of grated carrots
- 2 tbsp olive oil
- 1 tbsp lemon juice
- ½ tsp salt
- ¼ tsp black pepper
- ½ tsp mustard (Dijon or regular)
- ¼ tsp honey
- 2 tbsp chopped fresh seasonal herbs (parsley, marjoram, etc.)

Method
1. Whisk together the olive oil, lemon juice, mustard, honey, salt, black pepper, and herbs.
2. Grate the carrots and then mix into the dressing.

CELERIAC (CELERY ROOT) SALAD

Gluten-free, nut-free, vegetarian

This is one of the few raw salads I serve in the winter. Celery root is also delicious cooked into soups or roasted, but it has a lovely, crisp, celery-like taste that is perfect raw. This salad does seem to be a hit with children, as our friend's children who are fussy eaters have devoured it! The salad should not be dry, so sometimes I make a little more dressing or stop adding the shredded celery when it seems exactly right. Celery root is cooling and clears Liver and Stomach heat. Mustard is warming and stimulates digestion. Walnuts nourish Kidney *Yang* and are a perfect winter nut.

Ingredients
- 2 small celery roots or 4 cups, shredded
- 1 cup of Greek yoghurt or sour cream
- 2½ tbsp mustard
- 2 tbsp lemon juice
- 1 apple
- 1 tsp salt
- Optional: ¼ cup of walnuts, chopped

Method
1. Combine the yoghurt or sour cream with the mustard, lemon juice, and salt.
2. Grate the apple and add to the yoghurt mixture.
3. Shred the celery root and immediately mix into the yoghurt mixture to prevent browning.
4. Add walnuts if using.

CROCK POT BEEF AND BEAN, OR ONLY BEAN, CHILI

Gluten-free, nut-free, vegetarian, vegan

The beans, carrots, and squash (you can substitute any squash on hand) are all so nourishing to the Spleen and Stomach. Beef tonifies *Qi* and Blood. The slow cooking time for this recipe infuses warmth into the dish and makes it easy to digest. Black and red beans nourish the Kidneys and chickpeas nourish both the Kidneys and Spleen *Qi*. Oregano, cumin, coriander, and paprika stimulate digestion, and basil loosens phlegm.

Ingredients

- 1½ cups of adzuki or kidney beans (1 x 15 oz can)
- 1½ cups of black beans (1 x 15 oz can)
- 1½ cups of chickpeas (1 x 15 oz can)
- 1–2 cups of ground beef (optional)
- 1 cup of tomato sauce
- 3 cups of vegetable or beef stock
- 2 carrots, chopped
- 1 cup of butternut squash, diced small
- 6–10 mushrooms (Shiitake, brown, or white, optional)
- 1 onion, chopped
- 1 clove of garlic, chopped
- 1 tbsp dried oregano
- 1 tbsp dried basil
- 1–2 tbsp chili powder
- 1 tsp cumin
- 1 tsp ground coriander
- 1 tsp paprika

Method

1. If using beef, brown it in a saucepan and drain away the fat.
2. Add all the ingredients to a slow cooker and stir.
3. Cook on low for 7–8 hours or on high for 5–6.

Toppings: Can top with grated cheese, sour cream, or Greek yoghurt.

HONEY AND GINGER WILD SALMON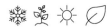

Gluten-free, nut-free

Salmon is a quick and relatively simple dinner to make. In the summer it can be paired with a light salad, and in the winter with grains and roasted vegetables for a heartier meal. Salmon is high in Omega-3 fatty acids, has a cooling thermal nature and nourishes *Qi* and Blood. The ginger will warm up the dish, benefit the Lungs, and warm the Middle Burner.

Ingredients

- 4 x 6 oz pieces of wild salmon
- ½ cup of honey
- ⅓ cup of soy sauce
- 2 tsp grated ginger

Method

1. Whisk the honey, soy sauce, and ginger together.
2. Marinate the salmon in half the mixture in the refrigerator for 15 minutes to a few hours or all day.
3. Preheat the oven to a high broil setting.
4. Place the salmon, skin side down, onto parchment paper.
5. Heat the remaining marinade in a small saucepan. Bring to a boil then reduce to simmer for 4 minutes. Remove and allow it to cool; it will thicken.
6. Broil the salmon for 8–12 minutes depending on thickness. It will continue to cook slightly when removed from the oven. Salmon should be flaky when done.
7. Pour the glaze over the salmon.

LEEK AND POTATO SOUP

Gluten-free, nut-free, vegetarian, vegan (use olive oil)

Classic yet simple, and easily gobbled up by the children. Wonderful as an accompaniment to dinner, a stand-alone lunch, or packed in a thermos for school. Leeks are warm and pungent and can be used at the first signs of a cold or flu with chills. Leeks nourish Kidney *Yang* and warm the digestion, helping with appetite and abdominal pain. They are available year-round but are best eaten in the fall, winter, and spring.

Ingredients

- 2 tbsp butter (can substitute with olive oil)
- 1 small onion (or ½ large onion), chopped
- 12 small Yukon gold potatoes or 4–5 Russet potatoes cut into ½ inch pieces
- 3–4 leeks, roughly chopped, rinsed very well
- 5–7 cups of water (can also use homemade stock or 2 bouillon cubes dissolved in the water)
- 2 bay leaves
- 3 sprigs of thyme
- 1 tsp salt (omit if using bouillon cubes)

Method

1. Melt the butter in a saucepan over a medium to low heat.
2. Sauté the onion for a few minutes.

3. Add the leeks and potatoes and continue to sauté for another 5–10 minutes until the vegetables have softened.
4. Add water or stock.
5. Add the bay leaves, thyme, and salt to the saucepan.
6. Turn up the heat, bring to a boil, and then reduce to low to simmer for 30–40 minutes.
7. Use a hand blender to blend until smooth.

LENTIL DAL

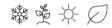

Gluten-free, nut-free, vegetarian, vegan

I often make dal in the pressure cooker and it is ready in under 30 minutes. I serve it over rice, quinoa, or millet, which is also ready in under 20 minutes. Dal is perfect for next-day lunches and packs well. I sometimes add a dollop of sour cream or Greek yoghurt before serving. Lentils benefit Essence (*Jing*) of the Kidneys, and red lentils tonify Heart and Kidney *Qi*.

Ingredients
- 1 cup of red lentils
- 3 cups of water (I sometimes use bone broth)
- 2 tbsp olive oil
- ½ onion, chopped
- 1 cup of mixed vegetables, chopped
- 1 large tomato, chopped or 2 tbsp tomato paste (can omit)
- 1 tbsp fresh ginger, chopped
- 1 tsp ground coriander
- 1 tsp cumin
- 1 tsp turmeric
- ¼ tsp ground cardamom
- ¼ tsp cinnamon
- 1 tsp salt

Method
1. Sauté the onions in the olive oil for 5 minutes.
2. Add the vegetables and ginger and continue to sauté.
3. Add the tomato or tomato paste.
4. Rinse the lentils and add to the vegetables.

5. Add the spices and salt (add the salt after cooking if using pressure cooker).

6. If you are using a pressure cooker, put the lid on, and cook for 3 minutes with the pressure regulator rocking slowly.

7. Remove from the heat, let the pressure drop of its own accord. If you are not using a pressure cooker, bring to a low boil, then reduce the heat to a simmer for 20 minutes.

8. You can cook this for longer in the fall and winter months.

MILLET (SIDE DISH)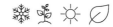
Gluten-free, nut-free, vegetarian, vegan

All the benefits listed above; it can also be served as an alternative to rice.

Ingredients
- 1 cup of millet
- 2 cups of water
- ½ tsp salt (optional)
- 2 tbsp butter or oil (optional)

Method
1. Toast the millet over a medium to high heat in saucepan for a few minutes to brown.
2. Add the water and salt and stir.
3. Bring to a boil, then cover and reduce to a simmer for 20 minutes.
4. Remove from the heat and let sit for 10 minutes.
5. Fluff with a fork and add butter or oil as desired.

MILLET SALAD
Gluten-free, nut-free, vegetarian, vegan

Leftover millet is perfect for school lunches. I always make extra when cooking it up as a side dish and it is best used in a salad the next day. The greens can be whatever you have on hand and are great for supporting the Liver. Parsley is pungent and helps with the upward and outward movement of spring. Black beans add protein, folate, iron, and fiber, tonify the Kidneys and are warming; this creates balance in the recipe as the cucumber, mint, and lemon juice are cold in nature.

Ingredients
- 2 cups of leftover cooked millet
- 1 tbsp parsley, finely chopped
- ½ tbsp mint, finely chopped
- 1 cup of Swiss chard or kale (sautéed on a high heat for a short time), spinach or lightly steamed asparagus (whatever the children are currently actually eating)
- 1 cup of black beans, cooked
- 1 cup of cucumber, diced

For the dressing:
- 3 tbsp lemon juice
- 2 tbsp olive oil
- ¼ tsp garlic powder
- Salt and pepper to taste

Method
1. For the dressing, whisk together the lemon juice, olive oil, garlic powder and about 1 tsp salt and ¼ tsp pepper.
2. In a separate bowl combine the millet, parsley, mint, choice of cooked greens, black beans, and cucumber. Mix well.
3. Add the dressing to the salad and mix in.
4. Taste and add salt and pepper as needed.
5. Let sit for at least 30 minutes before serving.

MILLET SOUPY PORRIDGE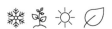
Gluten-free, nut-free, vegetarian, vegan

Millet is regarded as a highly nutritious healing food in TCM. It is a gluten-free grain and wonderful for children as it is extremely easy to digest. This porridge is also soothing for morning sickness and post-partum recovery. It can be served in the morning with the addition of raisins, seeds, nuts, cinnamon, dates, goji berries, fruit that is in season, maple syrup, or honey. Alternatively, it can be served alongside lunch or dinner as a nutritious accompaniment. It is bland and wonderful at harmonizing the digestion to stimulate the appetite, strengthening the Kidneys, and nourishing Blood and *Qi*. Serve to children regularly as their digestive systems will benefit greatly.

Ingredients

- ⅓ cup of millet, rinsed
- 6 cups of water

Method

1. Cover the millet with water in a saucepan.
2. Bring to a boil, and then reduce to a simmer for 30 minutes.
3. Stir occasionally to prevent the millet from sticking to the bottom of the pan.
4. For a thicker porridge, continue to cook for 10–30 more minutes.

ORANGE CHICKEN (OR TOFU) AND ALMONDS[10]

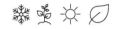

Gluten-free, vegetarian

This has been a favorite in the family for a long time. I cooked it for my children, who christened it "Orange Chicken," and now I cook it for my grandchildren. It is my sort of dish because you do not have to get the proportions exactly right. A dash of this and a splash of that is my style. It is quick and easy, the only thing worth mentioning is that it is really worth having EVERYTHING ready before you start. I cook it with chicken less often now because the chickens have changed. The only chickens I can find are new modern varieties that are so heavy that they cannot stand up without breaking their legs—and they don't have much taste. I have therefore developed a tofu version. (Julian Scott)

Chickens nourish *Qi* and Blood. Tofu benefits the Lungs and Large Intestine, and boosts and harmonizes the digestion.

Ingredients

- 1 lb chicken breasts or tofu
- White of an egg
- A knob of ginger
- Oil for frying
- A handful of flaked almonds (about 2 cups)
- 1 tbsp butter or 1 tbsp oil
- 2 tbsp soy sauce

---

10 Recipe generously submitted from Julian Scott, author of *Acupuncture in the Treatment of Children* and the world's most eminent pediatric acupuncture specialist who has been treating children with Chinese Medicine for over 40 years.

- 2 tbsp tomato paste
- 1 heaped tbsp corn flour mixed with ½ to ¾ cup of water

Method

1. Beat the egg white in a medium-sized bowl until it is runny.
2. Grate the ginger into the egg white.
3. Cut the chicken or tofu into ½ inch bits and stir into the ginger and egg white mix; leave to marinade for as long as is convenient.
4. Toast the flaked almonds until they are slightly browned. You can either do this in the oven or dry fry them. This is the only tricky bit, as it is easy to burn just a few of the flakes while the others are hardly warm. The secret is to heat the pan slowly and keep stirring. The moment you take your attention off them they will burn!
5. When you are ready to cook, using a heavy-based frying pan, fry the chicken very quickly in batches, to sear it. Poor quality chicken will ooze lots of water, so this will have to done in smaller batches. Tofu version: if the tofu is crumbly you can miss this stage, but if you have very rubbery tofu, pre-frying can improve the flavor.
6. Remove the chicken (or tofu) from the pan.
7. Melt the butter, add the tomato paste and mix it together; add the soy sauce and stir together for a few moments, then toss in the almond flakes.
8. Stir it around for a while until the almond flakes are covered, and then add the chicken or tofu.
9. Stir rapidly on a high heat, and then add the corn flour and water mix water for a satisfying sizzle.
10. Bring it slowly to a boil and keep it just boiling for a few minutes. (Watch that it does not burn.)
11. You can serve this with rice.

PEAS (SIDE DISH)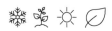
Gluten-free, nut-free, vegetarian, vegan

Peas are an easily loved vegetable by children and will not create any imbalances if eaten year-round. They have a neutral thermal nature and tonify the Spleen and Stomach and harmonize the digestion. They benefit the Liver and are beneficial to eat in the spring. They can be added as they are to lunches and stir fries, eaten as a side dish for lunch and dinner, added to macaroni and cheese, and mashed for younger children.

Ingredients
- 3 cups of fresh peas or frozen peas
- Butter or oil
- Dried or fresh seasonal herbs

Method
1. For fresh peas, steam in a vegetable steamer for 10 minutes, or bring to a boil in 1 tbsp water, reduce the heat and simmer for less than 5 minutes. Add butter and ½ tsp dried or 1 tsp fresh seasonal herbs: basil, thyme, mint, oregano, marjoram, rosemary, or chives.
2. For frozen peas, sauté for 3 minutes in 2 tbsp butter or oil over a medium to high heat, or bring to a boil in 1 tbsp water, reduce the heat and simmer for less than 5 minutes. Add ½ tsp dried or 1 tsp fresh seasonal herbs: basil, thyme, mint, oregano, marjoram, rosemary, or chives.

PESTO D'URTICA

Gluten-free, nut-free (use sunflower seeds), vegetarian, vegan (use nutritional yeast)

Nettles are a forager's dream—easy to identify and nutritionally worth it. Unsure if it is nettle? A quick poke at the plant and the sting left behind will assure you. Nettles are a wonderful remedy for spring allergies as they dispel wind and damp. They are cooling, as is lemon juice. Nettles are a *Yin* tonic and help to nourish blood. Gloves are needed to harvest, however, and only the tender tops taken off (2–3 leaf sets down from the top). Once steamed or boiled, they are ready to be eaten. This pesto can be enjoyed over noodles, in a sandwich, as a dip, or to dress a burger. Sunflower seeds can be substituted for the walnuts or pine nuts when using in school lunches.

Ingredients
- 1½ cups of steamed or boiled nettles (just over 1 cup of fresh nettles)
- 4 tbsp lemon juice
- ½–¾ cup of olive oil
- 1 tsp sea salt
- 3–4 tbsp Parmesan cheese, grated (can substitute with nutritional yeast)

  - ½ cup of walnuts or pine nuts (can substitute with sunflower seeds)
  - 1 clove of garlic
  - ½ cup of water (or more if needed)

Method

1. Prepare some iced water to cool the nettles after simmering.
2. With gloves, remove the nettle leaves from the stems and discard.
3. Bring a large saucepan of salted water to a simmer and add the nettles.
4. Stir for 30 seconds, drain in a colander, and immediately add to the iced water.
5. Drain the water and wring out excess water from the nettles.
6. Pulse the nuts or seeds, garlic, lemon juice, and salt in food processor.
7. Add the nettles and then pulse while slowly adding olive oil through the feed tube.
8. Add the Parmesan cheese and pulse a few more times.
9. Taste—you may need to add more salt.
10. This keeps for 5–7 days refrigerated or it can be frozen in an airtight container for future use.

STEAMED EGG SOUP[11]

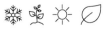

Gluten-free, nut-free

This is a nourishing recipe that Lillian Pearl Bridges makes for her grandchildren. Eggs nourish the Blood and *Yin*, they clear heat, and moisten the Lungs. Chicken broth nourishes Defensive *Qi* (*Wei Qi*) and benefits *Jing*. Sesame oil is cooling, moistening, and nourishes Kidney and Liver *Yin* and Blood.

Ingredients

  - 1 large egg
  - ½ cup of chicken broth
  - 1 tsp tamari or soy sauce
  - $^1/_4$ tsp sesame oil

Method

1. Whisk the egg and chicken broth together until light and frothy.

---

11 Recipe generously submitted from Lillian Pearl Bridges, author of *Face Reading in Chinese Medicine*.

2. Pour into a small heatproof rice bowl and place into an already hot steamer.
3. Steam for 12 minutes.
4. Remove carefully and pour the tamari or soy sauce and sesame oil over the egg.

SWEET POTATO AND BUTTER BEAN (LIMA BEAN) SOUP

Gluten-free, nut-free, vegetarian, vegan

Sweet potatoes are a wonderfully nourishing food for children. Easy to digest and strengthening to the Middle Burner, they nourish *Qi*, and tonify Kidney *Yin*. Butter beans are cooling, sweet, and benefit the Liver and Lungs.

Ingredients
- 2 medium sweet potatoes (or yams), cubed
- 3 cups of butter beans, cooked (2 x 15 oz cans)
- ½ cup of butter or olive oil
- 1 onion, chopped
- 5 cups of broth (vegetable or chicken)
- $^1/_5$ tsp black pepper
- 2–3 tsp cinnamon
- 1–2 tsp nutmeg
- 1 tsp salt

Method
1. Sauté the onion in oil or butter for a few minutes.
2. Add the sweet potatoes (or yams) and spices, salt, and pepper, and continue to sauté for 10 minutes.
3. Add a little broth to prevent sticking, then add the rest of the broth and mix.
4. Bring to a boil, reduce, and simmer for about 45 minutes.
5. If using a pressure cooker, set to the required setting for sweet potato (usually about 3–5 minutes).
6. When the sweet potatoes are cooked, add the butter beans and use a handheld blender to blend.
7. This makes a lot of soup, and can be used for lunches, etc.

VEGETARIAN LASAGNA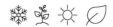
Nut-free, vegetarian

A versatile dish as the vegetables can be rotated depending on the season. The base of carrots, leeks, cabbage, and onion can stay consistent as these are year-round vegetables. The greens can be changed—spinach in the spring, arugula in the summer, and chard, kale, or collard greens in the winter. Carrots nourish the Spleen and Stomach. Leeks help to move Qi and nourish Kidney *Yang*. Cabbage balances the Spleen and Stomach. Onions move Qi and loosen phlegm.

Ingredients
- 3 carrots, diced
- 1 leek, chopped
- 1 cup of cabbage, chopped
- 1 yellow onion, chopped
- 2 tbsp olive oil
- 2 cups of greens (seasonal), chopped
- 2 cups of tomato sauce (to make: 2 cups of pureed tomatoes, ½ tsp salt, 2 tbsp olive oil, 2 tsp dried basil, 2 tsp rosemary, chopped)
- About 2 cups of ricotta cheese
- 1 tsp salt
- 2 tbsp fresh oregano and thyme leaves or 2 tsp dried
- ¼ tsp pepper
- 9 lasagna sheets
- 2 cups of grated cheese

Method
1. Preheat the oven to 425°F.
2. Sauté the carrots, leek, cabbage, and onion in olive oil for 10 minutes.
3. If making the tomato sauce, heat the ingredients in a saucepan and stir together.
4. Add the greens to the vegetable mix and mix in; let wilt for about 3 minutes.
5. Take half the ricotta and blend in a food processor. Remove and transfer to a bowl.
6. In the same food processor (don't rinse), add the cooked vegetables. Pulse a few times until they are more finely chopped but not mushy. Transfer to the bowl with the ricotta.
7. Add the remaining ricotta to the mixture. Add salt, pepper, and the herbs.

8. In a lasagna baking dish, spread ¼ of the tomato sauce, then layer 3 lasagna sheets, top this with half the vegetable/ricotta mixture, then ¼ of the tomato sauce, then ¼ of the grated cheese, 3 more lasagna sheets, the rest of the vegetable/ricotta mixture, then ¼ of the tomato sauce, ¼ of the grated cheese, top with 3 more lasagna sheets, the remaining tomato sauce, and the rest of the grated cheese.
9. Cover with parchment or foil and bake for 18 minutes.
10. Remove the covering and bake for an additional 12 minutes.
11. Let cool for 10–15 minutes before serving.

WATERMELON AND FETA SUMMER SALAD

Gluten-free, nut-free, vegetarian

This salad is refreshing and cooling—perfect for hot summer days. Make extra so it can be packed into a child's lunchbox. Watermelon has a cold thermal nature, clears heat, quenches thirst, and relieves irritability from summer heat. Because watermelon is cold in nature, it is not recommended for weak digestion and less is more for children. Sheep feta is recommended due to its creaminess, but any type will work. Sheep feta is warming, and mint leaves are cooling and promote sweating. Children should only have a small amount of this salad to protect their Middle Burners.

Ingredients
- About 5 cups of watermelon cubed into 1 inch pieces
- 1 cup of sheep feta
- 3 tbsp olive oil
- 1 tbsp lime juice
- ¼ cup of fresh mint leaves
- ½ tsp salt
- ¼ tsp pepper

Method
1. Chop the watermelon and place into a colander while mixing the rest of the ingredients.
2. In a small bowl whisk the olive oil, lime juice, salt, and pepper.
3. Add the watermelon to a salad bowl, pour the dressing over and throw over the mint leaves.
4. Mix gently.
5. Add the crumbled feta and toss gently.

Bibliography

Aatsinki, A.-K., Keskitalo, A., Laitinen, V., Munukka, E., *et al.* (2020) 'Maternal prenatal psychological distress and hair cortisol levels associated with infant fecal microbiota composition at 2.5 months of age.' *Psychoneuroendocrinology 119*, 104754.

Abrahamsson, T.R., Jakobsson, H.E., Andersson, A.F., Bjørkstén, B., Engstrand, L., and Jenmalm, M.C. (2014) 'Low gut microbiota diversity in early infancy precedes asthma at school age.' *Clinical & Experimental Allergy 44*, 6, 842–850.

AHA (American Heart Association) (2020) 'Healthy eating behaviors in childhood may reduce the risk of adult obesity and heart disease.' *ScienceDaily*, May 11.

Aitbali, Y., Ba-M'hamed, S., Elhidar, N., Nafis, A., Soraa, N., and Bennis, M. (2018) 'Glyphosate based-herbicide exposure affects gut microbiota, anxiety and depression-like behaviors in mice.' *Neurotoxicology and Teratology 67*, 44–49.

Akamatsu, R., Hasegawa, S., Ito, N., and Izumi, B.T. (2019) 'Gratitude for food may help to decrease food dislikes in children.' *Journal of Nutrition Education and Behavior 57*, 7, S110.

Andersson, N.W., Hansen, M.V., Larsen, A.D., Hougaard, K.S., Kolstad, H.A., and Schlünssen, V. (2016) 'Prenatal maternal stress and atopic diseases in the child: A systematic review of observational human studies.' *Allergy 71*, 1, 15–26.

Andrews, D. (no date) 'Rate Your Plate Series: Natural vs. Artificial Flavors.' 29 October. Available at: www.ewg.org/agmag/2014/10/synthetic-ingredients-natural-flavors-and-natural-flavors-artificial-flavors

Asha'ari, Z.A., Ahmad, M.Z., Jihan, W.S., Che, C.M., and Leman, I. (2013) 'Ingestion of honey improves the symptoms of allergic rhinitis: Evidence from a randomized placebo-controlled trial in the East coast of Peninsular Malaysia.' *Annals of Saudi Medicine 33*, 5, 469–475.

Ashkin, E. and Mounsey, A. (2013) 'PURLs: A spoonful of honey helps a coughing child sleep.' *The Journal of Family Practice 6*, 145–147.

Avern, R. (2019) *Acupuncture for Babies, Children and Teenagers: Treating Both the Illness and the Child.* London: Singing Dragon.

Bain, A.R., Lesperance, N.C., and Jay, O. (2012) 'Body heat storage during physical activity is lower with hot fluid ingestion under conditions that permit full evaporation.' *Acta Physiologica (Oxford) 206*, 2, 98–108.

Barker, D.J.P. (1990) 'The fetal and infant origins of adult disease.' *BMJ 301*, November. Available at: www.ncbi.nlm.nih.gov/pmc/articles/PMC1664286/pdf/bmj00206-0007.pdf

Barker, D.J.P. and Martyn, C.N. (1992) 'The maternal and fetal origins of cardiovascular disease.' *Journal of Epidemiology and Community Health 46*, 1, 8–11. doi:10.1136/jech.46.1.8.

Bayer, S.B., Gearry, R.B., and Drummond, L.N. (2018) 'Putative mechanisms of kiwifruit on maintenance of normal gastrointestinal function.' *Critical Reviews in Food Science and Nutrition 58*, 14, 2432–2452.

Bédard, A., Northstone, K., Henderson, J., and Shaheen, S.O. (2017) 'Maternal intake of sugar during pregnancy and childhood respiratory and atopic outcomes.' *European Respiratory Journal 50*, 1, 1700073.

Bielski, Z. (2009) 'Stress during pregnancy may lower baby's IQ.' The *Globe and Mail*, July 5. Available at: www.theglobeandmail.com/life/parenting/stress-during-pregnancy-may-lower-babys-iq/article597123

Blaabjerg, S., Artzi, D.M. and Aabenhus, R. (2017) 'Probiotics for the prevention of antibiotic-assisted diarrhea in outpatients—A systematic review and meta-analysis.' *Antibiotics (Basel) 6*, 4, 21.

Boney, C.M., Verma, A., Tucker, R., and Vohr, B.R. (2005) 'Metabolic syndrome in childhood: Association with birth weight, maternal obesity, and gestational diabetes mellitus.' *Pediatrics 115*, 3, e290–296.

Boyer, J.L. and Liu, R.H. (2004) 'Apple phytochemicals and their health benefits.' *Nutrition Journal 3*, 5.

Brannigan, R., Tanskanen, A., Huttunen, M.O., Cannon, M., Leacy, F.P. and Clarke, M.C. (2020) 'The role of prenatal stress as a pathway to personality disorder: Longitudinal birth cohort study.' *The British Journal of Psychiatry 216*, 2, 85–89.

Burton, G.J., Fowden, A.L., and Thornburg, K.L. (2016) 'Placental origins of chronic disease.' *Physiological Reviews 96*, 4, 1509–1565. doi:10.1152/physrev.00029.2015.

Cantrell, E. (2012) *40 Days to Enlightened Eating: Journey to Optimal Weight, Health, Energy, and Vitality.* Carlsbad, CA: Balboa Press.

Cao, X., Laplante, D.P., Brunet, A., Ciampi, A., and King, S. (2014) 'Prenatal maternal stress affects motor function in 5½-year-old children: Project Ice Storm.' *Developmental Psychobiology 56*, 1, 117–125.

Center on the Developing Child (2010) *The Foundations of Lifelong Health Are Built in Early Childhood.* Cambridge, MA: Center on the Developing Child, Harvard University. Available at: www.developingchild.harvard.edu

Chang, H.-H., Chen, C.-S., and Lin, J.-Y. (2012) 'Protective effect of dietary perilla oil on allergic inflammation in asthmatic mice.' *European Journal of Lipid Science and Technology 114*, 9, 1007–1015.

Chelimo, C., Camargo, C.A., Jr, Morton, S.M.B. and Grant, C.C. (2020) 'Association of repeated antibiotic exposure up to age 4 years with body mass at age 4.5 years.' *JAMA Network Open 3*, 1, e1917577.

Chien, L.Y., Tai, C.-J., Ko, Y.-L., Huang, C.-H., and Sheu, S.-J. (2006) 'Adherence to "Doing-the-month" practices is associated with fewer physical and depressive symptoms among postpartum women in Taiwan.' *Research in Nursing & Health 29*, 5, 374–383.

Crook, N., Ferreiro, A., Gasparrini, A.J., Pesesky, M.W., et al. (2019) 'Adaptive strategies of the candidate probiotic E. coli Nissle in the mammalian gut.' *Cell Host and Microbe*, 26 March. doi:10.1016/j.chom.2019.02.005.

Crossley, T.F., Griffith, R., Jin, W. and Lechene, V. (2018) 'A structural analysis of the decline of home-cooked food.' Available at: www.bc.edu/content/dam/bc1/schools/mcas/economics/pdf/seminars/CGJL.pdf

Davis, C.M. (1939) 'Results of the self-selection of diets by young children.' *Canadian Medical Association Journal 41*, 3, 257–261.

Deci, E.L., Koestner, R., and Ryan, R.M. (1999) 'A meta-analytic review of experiments examining the effects of extrinsic rewards on intrinsic motivation.' *Psychological Bulletin 125*, 6, 627–700.

De Filippis, F., Pellegrini, N., Vannini, L. and Jeffery, I.B. (2015) 'High-level adherence to a Mediterranean diet beneficially impacts the gut microbiota and associated metabolome.' *Gut 65*, 11.

Differding, M.K., Doyon, M., Bouchard, L., Perron, P., *et al.* (2020) 'Potential interaction between timing of infant complementary feeding and breastfeeding duration in determination of early childhood gut microbiota composition and BMI.' *Pediatric Obesity 15*, 8, e12642.

Duchesne, A., Liu, A., Jones, S.L., Laplante, D.P., and King, S. (2017) 'Childhood body mass index at 5.5 years mediates the effect of prenatal maternal stress on daughters' age at menarche: Project Ice Storm.' *Journal of Developmental Origins of Health and Disease 8*, 2, 168–177.

D'Vaz, N., Meldrum, S.J., Dunstan, J.A., Lee-Pullen, T.F., *et al.* (2012) 'Fish oil supplementation in early infancy modulates developing infant immune responses.' *Clinical and Experimental Allergy: Journal of the British Society for Allergy and Clinical Immunology 42*, 8, 1206–1216.

EAACI (The European Academy of Allergy and Clinical Immunology) (2015) *Advocacy Manifesto: Tackling the Allergy Crisis in Europe – Concerted Policy Action Needed.* Available at: www.eaaci.org/documents/EAACI_Advocacy_Manifesto.pdf

Eladak, S., Grisin, T., Moison, D., Guerquin, M.-J., *et al.* (2015) 'A new chapter in the bisphenol A story: Bisphenol S and bisphenol F are not safe alternatives to this compound.' *Fertility and Sterility 103*, 1, 11–21.

El Faki, T., Babikir, H.E., and Ali, K.E. (2001) 'Biochemical assessment of home made fluids and their acceptability in the management of diarrhea in children in the gezira state, Sudan.' *Journal of Family & Community Medicine 8*, 3, 83–88.

El-Heneidy, A., Abdel-Rahman, M., Mihala, G., Ross, L.J., and Comans, T.A. (2018) 'Milk other than breast milk and the development of asthma in children 3 years of age. A Birth Cohort Study (2006–2011).' *Nutrients 10*, 11, 1798.

European Commission (2020) *Farm to Fork Strategy—For a Fair, Healthy and Environmentally-Friendly Food System.* Available at: https://ec.europa.eu/food/farm2fork_en

Fagan, J., Bohlen, L., Patton, S., and Klein, K. (2020) 'Organic diet intervention significantly reduces urinary glyphosate levels in US children and adults.' *Environmental Research 189*, 109898. doi:10.1016/j.envres.2020.109898.

Fall, T., Lundholm, C., Örtqvist, A.K., Fall, K., *et al.* (2015) 'Early exposure to dogs and farm animals and the risk of childhood asthma.' *JAMA Pediatrics 169*, 11, e153219.

Fallon Morell, S. and Cowan, T.S. (2013) *The Nourishing Traditions Book of Baby and Child Care.* Washington, DC: New Trends Publishing Inc.

Feehley, T., Plunkett, C.H., Bao, R., Choi Hong, S.M., *et al.* (2019) 'Healthy infants harbor intestinal bacteria that protect against food allergy.' *Nature Medicine 25*, 3, 448–453.

Finlay, B.B. and Arrieta, M.-C. (2016) *Let Them Eat Dirt: Saving Your Child from an Oversanitized World.* Vancouver, BC: Greystone Books Ltd.

Flaws, B. (1996) *Keeping Your Child Healthy with Chinese Medicine: A Parent's Guide to the Care and Prevention of Common Childhood Diseases.* Fletcher, NC: Blue Poppy Press.

Flaws, B. (1998) *The Tao of Healthy Eating: Dietary Wisdom According to Traditional Chinese Medicine.* Fletcher, NC: Blue Poppy Press.

Gaskin, I.M. (2003) *Ina May's Guide to Childbirth.* London: Penguin Random House.

Glover, V.O., O'Donnell, K.J., O'Connor, T.G., and Fisher, J. (2018) 'Prenatal maternal stress, fetal programming, and mechanisms underlying later psychopathology—A global perspective.' *Development and Psychopathology 30*, 3, 843–854.

Goldenberg, J.Z., Lytvyn, L., Steurich, J., Parkin, P., Mahant, S. and Johnston, B.C. (2015) 'Probiotics for the prevention of pediatric antibiotic-associated diarrhea.' *Cochrane Database of Systematic Reviews*. Available at: www.cochranelibrary.com/cdsr/doi/10.1002/14651858.CD004827.pub4/full

Government of Canada (2020) 'Pesticides and food safety.' Available at: www.canada.ca/en/health-canada/services/about-pesticides/pesticides-food-safety.html

Grimm, K.A., Kim, S.A., Yaroch, A.L., and Scanlon, K.S. (2014) 'Fruit and vegetable intake during infancy and early childhood.' *Pediatrics 134*, Supplement 1, S63–S69.

Harbec, M.J. and Pagani, L.S. (2018) 'Associations between early family meal environment quality and later well-being in school-age children.' *Journal of Developmental and Behavioral Pediatrics 39*, 2, 136–143.

Harris, A. and Seckl, J. (2011) 'Glucocorticoids, prenatal stress and the programming of disease.' *Hormones and Behaviour 59*, 3, 279–289.

Hawkins, J., Baker, C., Cherry, L., and Dunne, E. (2019) 'Black elderberry (Sambucus nigra) supplementation effectively treats upper respiratory symptoms: A meta-analysis of randomized, controlled clinical trials.' *Complementary Therapies in Medicine 42*, 361–365.

Herrick, K.A., Fryar, C.D., Hamner, H.C., Park, S., and Ogden, C.L. (2019) 'Added sugars intake among US infants and toddlers.' *Journal of the Academy of Nutrition and Dietetics 120*, 1, 21–32.

Hibbeln, J.R., Spiller, P., Brenna, J.T., Golding, J., *et al.* (2019) 'Relationships between seafood consumption during pregnancy and childhood and neurocognitive development: Two systematic reviews.' *Prostaglandins, Leukotrienes and Essential Fatty Acids 151*, 14–36.

Hillier, T.A., Pedula, K.L., Schmidt, M.M., Mullen, J.A., Charles, M.-A., and Pettitt, D.J. (2007) 'Childhood obesity and metabolic imprinting: The ongoing effects of maternal hyperglycemia.' *Diabetes Care 30*, 9, 2287–2292.

Hobel, C.J., Goldstein, A., and Barrett, E.S. (2008) 'Psychosocial stress and pregnancy outcome.' *Clinical Obstetrics and Gynecology 51*, 2, 333–348.

Hodges, S.J. and Anthony, E.Y. (2012) 'Occult megarectum—A commonly unrecognized case of enuresis.' *Urology 79*, 2, 421–424.

Hsiao, Y.-C., Wang, J.-H., Chang, C.-L., Hsieh, C.-J., and Chen, M.-C. (2020) 'Association between constipation and childhood nocturnal enuresis in Taiwan: A population-based matched case-control study.' *BMC Pediatrics 20*, 35.

Hyland, C., Bradman, A., Gerona, R., Patton, S., *et al.* (2020) 'Organic diet intervention significantly reduces urinary glyphosate levels in US children and adults.' *Environmental Research 171*, 568–575.

Ingaramo, P., Alarcón, R., Muñoz-de-Toro, M., and Luque, E.H. (2020) 'Are glyphosate and glyphosate-based herbicides endocrine disruptors that alter female fertility?' *Molecular and Cellular Endocrinology*, 110934.

Jin, M., Qian, Z., Yin, J., Xu, W., and Zhou, X. (2019) 'The role of intestinal microbiota in cardiovascular disease.' *Journal of Cellular and Molecular Medicine 23*, 4, 2343–2350.

Johnson, C. and Eccles, R. (2005) 'Acute cooling of the feet and the onset of common cold symptoms.' *Family Practice 22*, 6, 608–613.

Jornayvaz, F.R., Vollenweider. P., Bochud, M., Mooser, V., Waeber, G., and Marques-Vidal, P. (2016) 'Low birth weight leads to obesity, diabetes and increased leptin levels in adults: The CoLaus study.' *Cardiovascular Diabetology 15*, 73.

Kastner, J. (2003) *Chinese Nutrition Therapy: Dietetics in Traditional Chinese Medicine (TCM) Second Edition.* Leipzig: Georg Thieme Verlag.

Kaul, E.A. (2019) 'Elevated fasting vs post-load glucose levels and pregnancy outcomes in gestational diabetes: A population-based study.' *Diabetic Medicine,* 114–122.

Keller, A., Litzelman, K., Wisk, L.E., Maddox, T., *et al.* (2012) 'Does the perception that stress affects health matter? The association with health and mortality.' *Health Psychology: Official Journal of the Division of Health Psychology, American Psychological Association 31,* 5, 677–684.

Khan, A.U., Jabeen, Q., and Gilani, A.H. (2011) 'Pharmacological basis for the medicinal use of cardamom in asthma.' *Bangladesh Journal of Pharmacology 6,* 1, 34–37.

Kim, Y.H., Kim, K.W., Lee, S.-Y., Koo, K.O., *et al.* (2019) 'Maternal perinatal dietary patterns affect food allergy development in susceptible infants.' *The Journal of Allergy and Clinical Immunology: In Practice 7,* 7, 2337–2347.

King, S. and Laplante, D.P. (2005) 'The effects of prenatal maternal stress on children's cognitive development: Project Ice Storm.' *Stress 8,* 1, 35–45.

Kinney, A. (no date) 'Ancient China.' In *Children and Youth in History,* Item #187. Available at: http://chnm.gmu.edu/cyh/items/show/187

Klingberg, S., Brekke, H.K., and Ludvigsson, J. (2019) 'Introduction of fish and other foods during infancy and risk of asthma in the All Babies in Southeast Sweden cohort study.' *European Journal of Pediatrics 178,* 3, 395–402.

Lange, K., Buerger, M., Stallmach, A. and Bruns, T. (2016) 'Effects of antibiotics on gut microbiota.' *Digestive Diseases (Basel) 34,* 3, 260–268.

Laplante, D.P., Brunet, A., Schmitz, N., Ciampi, A., and King, S. (2008) 'Project Ice Storm: Prenatal maternal stress affects cognitive and linguistic functioning in 5½-year-old children.' *Journal of the American Academy of Child & Adolescent Psychiatry 47,* 9, 1063–1072.

Lautarescu, A., Pecheva, D., Nosarti, C., Nihouam, J., *et al.* (2019) 'Maternal prenatal stress is associated with altered uncinate fasciculus microstructure in premature neonates.' *Biological Psychiatry 87,* 6, 559–569.

Lavelle, F., Spence, M., Hollywood, L., McGowan, L., *et al.* (2016) 'Learning cooking skills at different ages: A cross-sectional study.' *International Journal of Behavioral Nutrition and Physical Activity 13,* 1, 119.

Leboyer, F. (1999) *Loving Hands: The Traditional Art of Baby Massage.* New York: Newmarket Press.

Leggett, D. (1999) *Recipes for Self-Healing.* Torquay: Meridian Press.

Leggett, D. (2008) *Helping Ourselves: A Guide to Traditional Chinese Food Energetics.* Torquay: Meridian Press.

Leung, D.Y.M., Calatroni, A., Zaramela, L.S., LeBeau, P.K., *et al.* (2019) 'Cracks in the skin of eczema patients promote allergic diseases: Protecting and moisturizing the skin may help prevent food allergies, asthma and hay fever.' *National Jewish Health 11,* 480.

Li, S. (2009) 'On the fetal education of Han Dynasty.' *Journal of Xianyang Normal University,* 23–25.

Liu, J. and Schelar, E. (2012) 'Pesticide exposure and child neurodevelopment: Summary and implications.' *Workplace Health & Safety 60,* 5, 235–243.

Lu, H.C. (1986) *Chinese System of Food Cures: Prevention and Remedies.* New York: Sterling Publishing.

Maciocia, G. (1982) *Classic of Categories (Lei Jing).* Beijing: People's Health Publishing House, Beijing (first published 1624).

Maciocia, G. (1989) *The Foundations of Chinese Medicine.* London: Churchill Livingstone.

Maciocia, G. (1998) *Obstetrics and Gynecology in Chinese Medicine.* London: Elsevier Ltd, Section 6, 447–449.

Magnusson, J., Ekström, S., Kull, I., Håkansson, N., *et al.* (2017) 'Polyunsaturated fatty acids in plasma at 8 years and subsequent allergic disease.' *The Journal of Allergy and Clinical Immunology 142*, 2, P510–P516.

Mao, J., Jain, A., Denslow, N.D., Nouri, M.-Z., *et al.* (2020) 'Bisphenol A and bisphenol S disruptions of the mouse placenta and potential effects on the placenta–brain axis.' *PNAS: Proceedings of the National Academy of Sciences of the United States of America 117*, 9, 4642–4652.

Mao, Q., Manservisi, F., Panzacchi, S., Mandrioli, D., *et al.* (2018) 'The Ramazzini Institute 13-week pilot study on glyphosate and Roundup administered at human-equivalent dose to Sprague Dawley rats: Effects on the microbiome.' *Environmental Health 17*, 1, 50.

Maoshing Ni, P. (1995) *The Yellow Emperor's Classic of Medicine.* Boston, MA: Shambhala.

Martino, J.V., van Limbergen, J., and Cahill, L.E. (2017) 'The role of carrageenan and carboxymethylcellulose in the development of intestinal inflammation.' *Frontiers in Pediatrics 5*, 96.

McClure, V. (1997) *The Tao of Motherhood.* Novato, CA: New World Library.

McGonigal, K. (2016) *The Upside of Stress.* London: Vermilion.

Mennella, J.A. and Bobowski, N.K. (2015) 'The sweetness and bitterness of childhood: Insights from basic research on taste preferences.' *Physiology & Behavior 152*, 502–507.

Mennella, J.A., Jagnow, P.C., and Beauchamp, G.K. (2001) 'Prenatal and postnatal flavor learning by human infants.' *Pediatrics 107*, 6, E88.

Mills, S., Brown, H., Wrieden, W., White, M., and Adams, J. (2017) 'Frequency of eating home cooked meals and potential benefits for diet and health: Cross-sectional analysis of a population-based cohort study.' *The International Journal of Behavioral Nutrition and Physical Activity 14*, 1, 109.

Monk, C., Lugo-Candelas, C. and Trumpff, C. (2019) 'Prenatal developmental origins of future psychopathology: Mechanisms and pathways.' *Annual Review of Clinical Psychology 15*, 1, 1–28.

Moore, J.B., Horti, A., and Fielding, B.A. (2018) 'Evaluation of the nutrient content of yogurts: A comprehensive survey of yogurt products in the major UK supermarkets.' *BMJ Open 8*, 8, e021387.

Nielsen, C.C., Gascon, M., Osornio-Vargas, A.R., Shier, C., *et al.* (2020) 'Natural environments in the urban context and gut microbiota in infants.' *Environment International 142.* Available at www.sciencedirect.com/science/article/pii/S0160412020318365?via%3Dihub

Osakabe, N., Takano, H., Sanbongi, C., Yasuda, A., *et al.* (2004) 'Anti-inflammatory and anti-allergic effect of rosmarinic acid (RA): inhibition of seasonal allergic rhinoconjunctivitis (SAR) and its mechanism.' *Biofactors 21*, 1–4, 127–131.

Painter, R.C., Osmond, C., Gluckman, P., Hanson, M., Phillips, D.I.W., and Roseboom, T.J. (2008) 'Transgenerational effects of prenatal exposure to the Dutch famine on neonatal adiposity and health in later life.' *BJOG: An International Journal of Obstetrics and Gynaecology 115*, 10, 1243–1249.

Pan, Y., Deng, M., Li, J., Du, B., *et al.* (2020) 'Occurrence and maternal transfer of multiple bisphenols, including an emerging derivative with unexpectedly high concentrations, in the human maternal-fetal-placental unit.' *Environmental Science & Technology 54*, 6, 3476–3486.

Patel, J. and Patel, P. (2019) 'Consequences of repression of emotion: Physical health, mental health and general well being.' *International Journal of Psychotherapy Practice and Research 1*, 3, 10.14302/issn.2574-612X.ijpr-18-2564.

Patrick, D.M., Sbihi, H., Dai, D.L.Y., Al Mamun, A., *et al.* (2020) 'Decreasing antibiotic use, the gut microbiota, and asthma incidence in children: Evidence from population-based and prospective cohort studies.' *The Lancet, Respiratory Medicine*, 24 March.

Paul, I.M., Beiler, J., McMonagle, A., Shaffer, M.L., Duda, L., and Berlin, C.M. (2007) 'Effect of honey, dextromethorphan, and no treatment on nocturnal cough and sleep quality for coughing children and their parents.' *Archives of Pediatrics & Adolescent Medicine* *161*, 12, 1140–1146.

Pitchford, P. (2002) *Healing with Whole Foods: Asian Traditions and Modern Nutrition* (3rd edn). London: Penguin Random House.

Pollan, M. (2007) *The Omnivore's Dilemma: A Natural History of Four Meals.* London: Penguin.

Provençal, N., Arloth, J., Cattaneo, A., Anacker, C., *et al.* (2019) 'Glucocorticoid exposure during hippocampal neurogenesis primes future stress response by inducing changes in DNA methylation.' *PNAS: Proceedings of the National Academy of Sciences of the United States of America 117*, 38, 23280–23285.

Pryde, S.E., Duncan, S.H., Hold, G.L., Stewart, C.S., and Flint, H.J. (2002) 'The microbiology of butyrate formation in the human colon.' *FEMS Microbiology Letters 217*, 2, 133–139.

Rakers, F., Rupprecht, S., Dreiling, M., Bergmeier, C., Witte, O.W. and Schwab, M. (2017) 'Transfer of maternal psychosocial stress to the fetus.' *Neuroscience and Biobehavioral Reviews* S0149–7634(16)30719–9.

Richardson, N. (2011) '*Translating Taijiao: Modern Metaphors and International Eclecticism in Song Jiazhao's Translation of Shimoda Jirō's Taikyō.*' *Research on Women in Modern Chinese History 19*, 255–288.

Rickman, J.C., Bruhn, C.M., and Barrett, D.M. (2007) 'Nutritional comparison of fresh, frozen, and canned fruits and vegetables II. Vitamin A and carotenoids, vitamin E, minerals and fiber.' *Journal of the Science of Food and Agriculture 87*, 1185–1196.

Robbins, K., Jacobs, M., Ramos, A., Balas, K., and Herbert, L. (2018) 'Prenatal food allergen avoidance practices for food allergy prevention.' *Annals of Allergy, Asthma & Immunology 121*, 5, S55–S56.

Rochester, J.R. and Bolden, A.L. (2015) 'Bisphenol S and F: A systematic review and comparison of the hormonal activity of bisphenol A substitutes.' *Environmental Health Perspectives 123*, 7, 643–650.

Rose, G. (1985) 'Sick individuals and sick populations.' *International Journal of Epidemiology 14*, 32–38.

Roseboom, T.J., van der Meulen, J.H., Ravelli, A.C., Osmond, C., Barker, D.J., and Bleker, O.P. (2001) 'Effects of prenatal exposure to the Dutch famine on adult disease in later life: An overview.' *Molecular and Cellular Endocrinology 185*, 1–2, 93–98.

Rueter, K., Jones, A.P., Siafarikas, A., Lim, E.-M., *et al.* (2019) 'Direct infant UV light exposure is associated with eczema and immune development.' *Journal of Allergy and Clinical Immunology 143*, 3, 1012–1020.

Rutherford, G. (2020) 'Living close to green space benefits gut bacteria of urban, formula-fed infants.' *ScienceDaily*, July 9. Available at: www.sciencedaily.com/releases/2020/07/200709135616.htm

Sampson, H. (2016) 'Anaphylaxis and emergency treatment.' *Pediatrics 111*, 6 Pt 3, 1601–1608.

Schab, D.W. and Trinh, N.-H.T. (2004) 'Do artificial food colors promote hyperactivity in children with hyperactive syndromes? A meta-analysis of double-blind placebo-controlled trials.' *Journal of Developmental and Behavioral Pediatrics 25*, 6, 423–434.

Scott, J. and Barlow T. (2018) *Acupuncture in the Treatment of Children Fourth Edition.* Halifax: Portway Press.

Shao, Y., Forster, S.C., Tsaliki, E., Vervier, K., *et al.* (2019) 'Stunted microbiota and opportunistic pathogen colonization in caesarean-section birth.' *Nature 574*, 117–121.

Sihui, H. (2015) *Principles of Correct Diet.* Zhengzhou: Zhongzhou Ancient Books Publishing House.

Simpson, H.L. and Campbell, B.J. (2015) 'Review article: Dietary fiber-microbiota interactions.' *Alimentary Pharmacology & Therapeutics 42*, 158–179.

Stearns, J.C., Simioni, J., Gunn, E., McDonald, H., *et al.* (2017) 'Intrapartum antibiotics for GBS prophylaxis after colonization patterns in the early infant gut microbiome of low risk infants.' *Scientific Reports 7*, 16527.

Stefka, A.T., Feehley, T., Tripathi, P., J. Qiu, J., *et al.* (2014) 'Commensal bacteria protect against food allergen sensitization.' *Proceedings of the National Academy of Sciences 111*, 36, 13145–13150.

Stein, A.D., Kahn, H.S., Rundle, A., Zybert, P.A., van der Pal-de Bruin, K., and Lumey, L.H. (2007) 'Anthropometric measures in middle age after exposure to famine during gestation: Evidence from the Dutch famine.' *The American Journal of Clinical Nutrition 85*, 3, March, 869–876. Available at: https://doi.org/10.1093/ajcn/85.3.869

Stephenson, J., Heslehurst, N., Hall, J., Schoenaker, D.A.J.M., *et al.* (2018) 'Before the beginning: Nutrition and lifestyle in the preconception period and its importance for future health.' *The Lancet 391*, 10132, 1830–1841.

Strauss, S. (2006) 'Clara M. Davis and the wisdom of letting children choose their own diets.' *CMAJ 175*, 10, 1199–1201.

Tabak, C., Wijga, A.H., de Meer, G., Janssen, N.A.H., Brunekreef, B., and Smith, H.A. (2006) 'Diet and asthma in Dutch school children.' *Thorax 61*, 12, 1048–1053.

The Lancet (2019) 'The Double Burden of Malnutrition.' December 16. Available at: www.thelancet.com/series/double-burden-malnutrition

Thurow, R. (2016) *The First 1000 Days: A Crucial Time for Mothers and Children and the World.* New York: PublicAffairs.

Torabian, G., Valtchev, P., Adil, Q., and Dehghani, F. (2019) 'Anti-influenza activity of elderberry (Sambucus nigra).' *Journal of Functional Foods 54*, 353–360.

Tryon, M.S., Carter, C.S., DeCant, R., and Laugero, K.D. (2013) 'Chronic stress exposure may affect the brain's response to high calorie food cues and predispose to obesogenic eating habits.' *Physiology & Behavior 120*, 233–242.

Tsakok, T., Marrs, T., Mohsin, M., Baron, S., *et al.* (2017) 'Does atopic dermatitis cause food allergy? A systematic review.' *The Lancet 137*, 4, 1071–1078.

Tun, H.M., Konya, T., Takaro, T.K., Brook, J.R., *et al.* (2017) 'Exposure to household furry pets influences the gut microbiota of infants at 3–4 months following various birth scenarios.' *Microbiome 5*, 40.

Turcotte-Tremblay, A.M., Lim, R., Laplante, D.P., Kobzik, L., Brunet, A., and King, S. (2014) 'Prenatal maternal stress predicts childhood asthma in girls: Project Ice Storm.' *BioMed Research International.* Available at: https://doi.org/10.1155/2014/201717

Tzu, L. (2018) *Tao Te Ching: The Essential Translation of the Ancient Chinese Book of the Tao* (J. Minford, Trans.). New York: Viking Press.

University of Calgary (2009) 'Early childhood diet may influence future health.' *ScienceDaily*, 15 January.

University of South Florida (USF Innovation) (2019) 'Gut microbiome of premature babies is associated with stunted growth. *ScienceDaily*, 4 November.

Utter, J., Larson, N., Laska, M.N., Winkler, M., and Neumark-Sztainer, D. (2018) 'Self-perceived cooking skills in emerging adulthood predict better dietary behaviors and intake 10 years later: A longitudinal study.' *Journal of Nutrition Education and Behavior 50*, 5, 494–500.

Valles-Colomer, M.F., Falony, G., Darzi, Y., Tigchelaar, E.F., *et al.* (2019) 'The neuroactive potential of the human gut microbiota in quality of life and depression.' *Nature Microbiology 4*, 623–632.

van de Loo, K.F.E., van Gelder, M.H.J., Roukema, J., Roeleveld, N., Merkus, J.F.M., and Verhaak, C.M. (2016) 'Prenatal maternal psychological stress and childhood asthma and wheezing: A meta-analysis.' *European Respiratory Journal 47*, 133–146.

Venekamp, R.P., Damoiseaux, R.A.M.J. and Schilder, A.G.M. (2014) 'Acute otitis media in children.' *BMJ Clinical Evidence*, 0301.

Venter, C., Maslin, K., Holloway, J.W., Silveira, L.J., *et al.* (2020) 'Different measures of diet diversity during infancy and the association with childhood food allergy in a UK birth cohort study.' *The Journal of Allergy and Clinical Immunology 8*, 6, P2017–P2026.

Veru, F., Dancause, K.N., Laplante, D.P., and King, S. (2015) 'Prenatal maternal stress predicts reductions in CD4+ lymphocytes.' *Physiology & Behavior 144*, 137–145.

Wang, B., Yao, M., Lv, L., Ling, Z., and Li, L. (2017) 'The human microbiota in health and disease.' *Engineering 3*, 1, 71–82.

Wassermann, B., Müller, H. and Berg, G. (2019) 'An apple a day: Which bacteria do we eat with organic and conventional apples?' *Frontiers in Microbiology* 10. doi:10.3389/fmicb.2019.01629.

Watt, J. and Marcus, R. (1973) 'Experimental ulcerative disease of the colon in animals.' *Gut 14*, 6, 506–510.

Weinstock, M. (2008) 'The long-term behavioural consequences of prenatal stress.' *Neuroscience & Biobehavioral Reviews 32*, 1073–1086.

Wilms, S. (2010) 'Nurturing life in classical Chinese Medicine: Sun Simiao on healing without drugs, transforming bodies, and cultivating life.' *Journal of Chinese Medicine 93*, 12.

Wilms, S. (2018) 'Nurturing the Foetus in Medieval China. Illustrating the 10 Months of Pregnancy.' In V. Lo and P. Barrett (eds) *Imagining Chinese Medicine* (pp.101–110). Leiden: Brill (Abridged, Illustrated Edition).

Wilms, S. and Betts, D. (no date) 'Nurturing the fetus.' Available at: https://healthyseminars.com/

Wilson, B. (2015) *First Bite: How We Learn to Eat*. New York: Basic Books.

Wong, H.B. (1981) 'Rice water in treatment of infantile gastroenteritis.' *The Lancet 2*, 8237, 102–103.

Wood, A.C., Blissett, J.M., Brunstrom, J.M., Carnell, S., *et al.* (2020) 'Caregiver influences on eating behaviors in young children: A scientific statement from the American Heart Association.' *Journal of the American Heart Association 9*, 10, e014520. doi:10.1161/JAHA.119.014520.

Wu, Y., Kapse, K., Jacobs, M., Niforatos-Andescavage, N., *et al.* (2020) 'Association of maternal psychological distress with in utero brain development in fetuses with congenital heart disease.' *JAMA Pediatrics*, e195316.

Zbuchea, A. (2014) 'Up-to-date use of honey for burns treatment.' *Annals of Burns and Fire Disasters 27*, 1, 22–30.

Zeinstra, G.G., Vrijhof, M., and Kremer, S. (2018) 'Is repeated exposure the holy grail for increasing children's vegetable intake? Lessons learned from a Dutch childcare intervention using various vegetable preparations.' *Appetite 121*, 316–325.

Zmora, N., Zilberman-Schapira, G., Suez, J., Halpern, Z., *et al.* (2018) 'Personalized gut mucosal colonization resistance to empiric probiotics is associated with unique host and microbiome features.' *Cell 174*, 6, P1388–P1405.

Index

CPI Antony Rowe
Eastbourne, UK
June 01, 2023